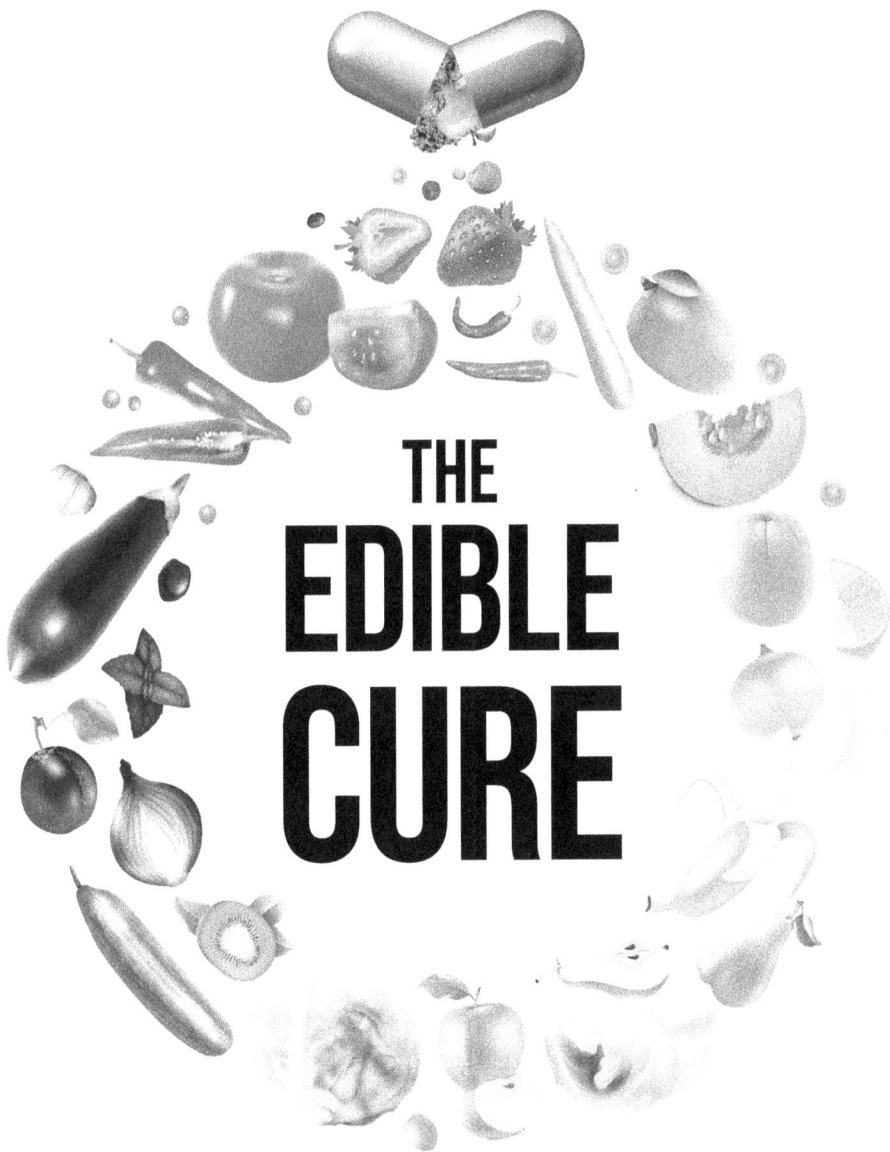

THE
EDIBLE
CURE

Foods That Heal from **A** to **Z**

KRISTINA GRANT

THE EDIBLE CURE: FOODS THAT HEAL FROM A TO Z

THE EDIBLE CURE: FOODS THAT HEAL
FROM A TO Z ©2020 Kristina Grant

ISBN-13: 978-0-578-66193-3

Published by Grant Wellness Publishing
Houston, TX

Printed in the United States of America
First Edition April 2020

Cover Design by Make Your Mark Publishing Solutions
Interior Layout by Make Your Mark Publishing Solutions
Editing by Make Your Mark Publishing Solutions

CONTENTS

Introduction xiii

A

Apples 2
Asparagus 3
Astragalus 5
Avocado 6
Apricots 8
Apple cider vinegar 9
Alpha Lipoic Acid 12
Aloe Vera 13
Artichoke 15

B

Bananas 18
Beets 19
Blueberries 20
Brussels sprouts 22
Broccoli 24
Bean Sprouts 25
Black Seed Oil 26
Berberine 29
Broccoli sprouts 30
Black Elderberry 32
Blackberries 35
Biotin 36

Banana peppers 37

Bok choy 38

Brazil nuts 41

C

Coffee 44

Carrots 45

Chia Seeds 46

Cantaloupe 48

Celery 50

Cherries 52

Cat's Claw 53

Cucumber 54

Cranberries 55

Chicory root 56

Cashews 57

Chlorella 59

Chaga Mushroom 60

D

Dates 64

Dragon Fruit 65

Dill 66

Dark Chocolate 67

E

Eggplants 70

Elm Bark 72

Egg 73

Edamame 74

Echinacea 75

F

Fennel 78
Fig...79
Fenugreek 80
Flaxseed 81

G

Grapefruit 86
Grapes..87
Guava...89
Ginseng.. 90
Ginger..92
Green Tea 93
Gingko...94

H

Honey 96
Hibiscus...98
Hackberry..99
Honeydew Melon...............................100
Hempseed 102

J

Jackfruit 106
Jicama 107
Jambolan..109
Jasmine 110
Juniper Berry 111
Jojoba...112

K

Kefir 116

Kiwi 118

Kumquat 120

Kale 121

L

Lychee 124

Lemon...125

Loquat 127

Longan..128

L-Lysine 129

Lutein 130

Lemongrass 131

Lavender 133

Lady's Mantle...135

Lungwort..136

Licorice Root 137

M

Mango 140

Mulberry...141

Milk Thistle..142

Melatonin 144

Manganese..145

N

Neem Oil..148

Nutmeg...149

Nectarines...150

Niacin 152

O

Olive Leaf 154
Oranges 156
Oats 158
Oakmoss 160
Onion 161
Oil of Oregano 163

P

Pineapple 166
Papaya 168
Pears 170
Palm Oil 172
Pumpkin 173
Prickly Pear 174
Potato (Sweet) 175
Peppermint 176
Pomegranate 178
Pine Bark 180
Passionflower 181
Parsley 182
Parsnip 184
Persimmon 185

Q

Quinoa 188
Quince 190

R

Raspberries 192
Rambutan 193

Rose Hips 194
Radish 195
Rosemary 196
Rhubarb 198
Resveratrol 199

S

Spirulina 202
Seaweed 204
Strawberries 206
Spinach 208
Sesame seeds 211
Safflower Oil 213
Saffron 214
Sage 215
Sunflower Lecithin 217
Stevia 218
Stone Root 219
St. John's Wort 220
Saw Palmetto 222
Spaghetti Squash 224
Star Fruit 225

T

Tomato 228
Tangerines 230
Tamarind 231
Tarragon 232
Tea Tree Oil 233
Thyme 234
Turmeric 236
Thiamine 238

U

Ugli fruit..240
Usnea..241

V

Vanilla Oil 244
Verbena...245
Valerian Root...246

W

Watermelon...250
Willow Bark...252
Wheat Bran..253
Wheatgrass 254

Y

Yogurt...258
Yucca.. 260
Yerba Santa 261
Yarrow...262

Z

Zucchini 264

Acknowledgments....................................269
Notes 273

INTRODUCTION

I've had a passion for health and nutrition from an early age. I did crunches in the den and daily workouts with fitness guru Gilad at the age of ten—crazy, right? As I grew older, my love for health turned into my career as a personal trainer with a BS in nutrition. Then it became my life as I practiced what I preached. Daily, people asked, "What do you eat?" "How can I lose weight?" or "I always workout and lose weight, but I can't get my stomach to go down. What should I do?" I found myself constantly giving advice and tips, and I easily became overwhelmed; I knew there had to be a more efficient way to reach people and answer their questions.

When my father was diagnosed with high cholesterol, the doctor wanted to put him on medication, but I convinced him to give me three months to change my father's diet, and if his low-density lipoproteins (LDL) numbers were not improved, he would start taking medicine. To this day, my father has never taken medication for high cholesterol, and he no longer has it. I wanted more people to know they could improve their lives and overall health by making small changes to their diet, but I wondered how I could reach the greatest amount of people and help them identify exactly what they need to eat. Then it hit me—write a book!

This book will not only help you, but it will also make a change in the world and how we view and approach food daily. Food is medicine, and when you change how you view it, you change your lifestyle. We will explore a variety of foods and their health benefits from A to Z. I hope this book educates and inspires you and, overall, makes you truly love eating real food!

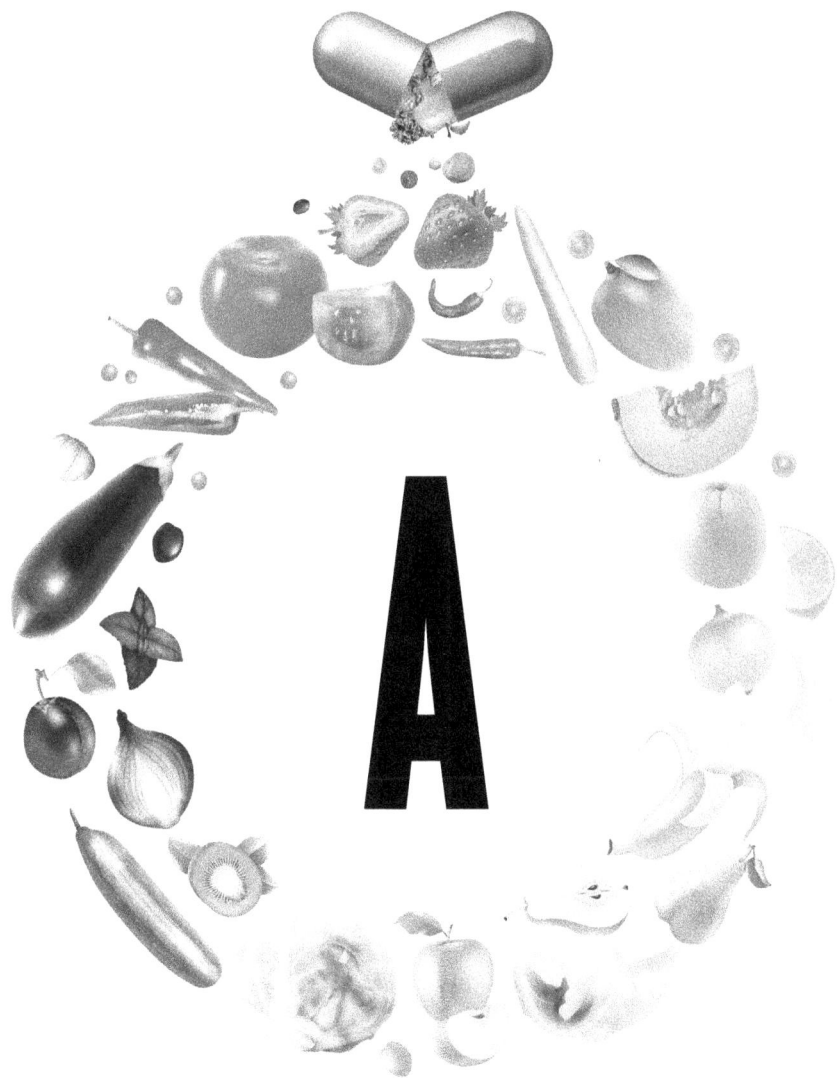

APPLES

For ages, we've heard "An apple a day keeps the doctor away," but what does that really mean? How do apples keep the doctor away? Well, apples are not just good to look at. There are thousands of types of apples, and they have great health benefits. Biting and chewing an apple stimulates saliva, therefore helping to prevent tooth decay by getting rid of bacteria. Apples are also full of pectin,[1] a soluble fiber that helps to prevent many health issues like free radicals, which are unstable atoms that cause stress and damage to our cells, and Parkinson's disease. They also prevent gallstones by ensuring there's not too much cholesterol in the bile, and they even help release stubborn stool. Pectin can lower cholesterol levels, help with diabetes by curving sugar levels, decrease your weight by making you feel fuller longer, and reduce the effects of irritable bowel syndrome (IBS).

Apples not only help with minor health problems, but also serious diseases and life-threatening diagnoses like cancers and liver disease. Scientists have shown that the consumption of apples can reduce the risk of developing cancer. In the apple peel are anti-growth properties that fight against cancer cells. The chances of developing liver, colon, breast, and pancreatic cancer can be reduced by eating apples.

Apples help detoxify the liver, decrease inflammation, and improve the heart. They also contain quercetin, which is an antioxidant that fortifies your immune system. Apples are good post-workout snacks with almond butter and can be used to make dessert for those late-night sweet cravings.

ASPARAGUS

Now, we're going to talk about the vegetable that makes your urine smell. Yeah, you know what it is—asparagus. Asparagus is a good source of fiber and contains essential vitamins and chromium, which enhances the ability of insulin to transport glucose from the bloodstream into the cells.

Asparagus is a natural diuretic, which promotes the production of urine, causing excretion of excess water from the body. It's good for individuals who suffer from edema, which is excess accumulation of fluid in the body and body tissues. For women who are prone to urinary tract infections (UTI), eating asparagus decreases the swelling, pain, and frequency of the infection.

Ever been in a rut sexually or just not in the mood? Try eating asparagus. It is a natural aphrodisiac because it contains folate and vitamin B6, which are known to enhance feelings of arousal. Asparagus can also stimulate estrogen and testosterone hormones due to the vitamin E it contains. All the more reason to eat this vegetable. "Let's Get It On!" But what if that one steamy night leads to pregnancy? Don't worry, asparagus can still benefit.

Asparagus contains about twenty-two percent of the recommended daily allowance of folate, which is crucial for pregnant women or women who want to become pregnant. Folate helps lower the chances of neural tube defects in the fetus. It also helps make new proteins and cells in the body, which is vital when developing a baby. It is also an excellent source of vitamin K, which helps reduce bone fractures by increasing your bone mineral density.

Do you take forever to stop bleeding when you get a cut? Not to worry; asparagus helps your blood clot, and it helps prevent atherosclerosis, which is the hardening of your arteries.

It is a good source of fiber because one serving contains more than a gram of soluble fiber, which helps soften stool, making digestion easier and smoother. High fiber intake means less chances of heart disease, congestive heart failure or (CHF), and type 2 diabetes. It also decreases the risk of obesity, high cholesterol, high blood pressure, hypertension, stroke, and much more. Many Americans don't take in nearly as much fiber as they should, so eating asparagus is an easy way to get that fiber in.

Asparagus has a significant amount of thiamine. *Great ... What does that mean?* Thiamine is a B vitamin, and it's crucial for the development of our bodies and our energy levels. It helps the body convert carbohydrates to energy. B vitamins help metabolize those donuts we love and the bread and pasta we intake to help us maintain balanced blood sugar.

Lastly, asparagus helps fight cancer. *How?* It contains glutathione. *Okay, what is that?* Glutathione is a compound that helps fight and destroy carcinogens. It is huge when it comes to protecting our healthy cells and regulating immune function.[2] So if your family is known to have bone, breast, lung and/or colon cancers, try making asparagus a staple in your diet to help lower your chances of developing it, too.

Wait, I've seen purple asparagus in the stores. What's the difference? Purple asparagus has slightly less fiber than green asparagus but has more protein and vitamin C. It's full of anthocyanins, which gives it its color and antioxidant effects that help fight damaging free radicals.

ASTRAGALUS

Astragalus? Never heard of it. Is it a plant? Well, yes and a root. Astragalus can lower your cholesterol and boost the immune system all because it has the active compound saponin. I know it's hard to pronounce, but you don't need to be able to pronounce it, just be able to ingest it to receive the benefits. Have a weak immune system and always sick? Astragalus helps prevent the common cold and flu. It also inhibits herpes, heals wounds, and lowers cortisol levels, all possible because flavonoids and polysaccharides are in astragalus. They're known to fight free radicals, prevent viruses and even have anti-inflammatory, antiviral, and antimicrobial capabilities.

I know you're wondering, *Can this plant really heal wounds and prevent the common cold?* Yes! It can control your helper T-cells, the cells that deal with the immune system and your fight or flight response. Furthermore, it can lower your blood pressure and triglycerides, which is imperative to a healthy heart and overall cardiovascular system. Are you insulin sensitive or resistant? Astragalus can help with diabetes and relieve insulin resistance by protecting pancreatic beta cells. From renal disease and kidney issues to cell regeneration and repair of tissues, astragalus can be life changing.

Even asthma may be reduced by taking astragalus. Inflammation in your lungs and airways and mucus can be lowered greatly, possibly decreasing the amount of attacks.

What about problems with the skin like scarring from dark marks? Astragalus can minimize scars, even if you have eczema or acute dermatitis like I do. It can help alleviate the inflammation and decrease your chances of scarring.

AVOCADO

Are avocados a vegetable or a fruit? They contain a seed, so technically, they are a fruit, even though they're viewed in society as a vegetable. Avocados are the number-one known source of healthy fats, but they provide numerous health benefits.

I have always heard people like Dr. Oz and others say avocado is a superfood, but how? Let's break down the different types of fats. Avocados contain "good" fat because they're made of mostly mono-unsaturated fats. These fats are known to be great for the heart. They help fight against atherosclerosis and aid in preventing unwanted plaque in the arterial walls and arteries.[3]

Also, avocados are high in fat-soluble vitamins such as vitamins K, A, and E, which are all necessary for proper body function and can impact our metabolic function as well. Avocados are packed with antioxidants and carotenoids, which are phytochemicals that aid our body in fighting against free radical damage and oxidative stress. The carotenoids make avocadoes great for our hair, to get that healthy shine we desire, and it promotes healthy skin. They are packed with protein to help repair damaged cells and hair follicles while providing enough protein for vegans and pescatarians who strive for sufficient protein intake.

Want a good face mask? Try mashing avocado in a bowl. (Add a little water for a looser texture.) They are great at reducing inflammation, brightening dark marks, and moisturizing your skin without harsh chemicals, leaving a radiant glow.

Did you know avocadoes are considered a low-sugar, high-fiber fruit? Suffer from constipation or irregular bowel movements? Avocadoes contain more than ten percent of our daily need of fiber and help coat the lining of the intestines to ease bowel movements and increase the frequency. More fiber helps add bulkiness to your stool and gives the sensation of satisfaction, meaning your appetite will likely decrease, aiding in weight loss.

Now, when you think of potassium, what is the first fruit that comes to mind? Bananas, right? Well, an avocado has double the amount of potassium as one banana. Looking for ways to boost your immune system heading into the fall and winter seasons? Avocadoes are full of vitamins B and C, which help your body combat unwanted illness and viruses and make copies of the viruses to prevent the illnesses from reoccurring. I wear glasses, and the eye doctor informed me that I am at risk for macular degeneration. But I learned avocadoes are great for vision health because they contain the carotenoid[4] lutein, which is known for taking in the light rays that could be damaging to the eyes, thereby lowering my chances of developing eye diseases such as cataracts and macular degeneration.

Now do you see why avocadoes are a superfood? From the fiber to potassium, heart health, and even eye benefits, avocadoes are an excellent fruit with endless health benefits.

APRICOTS

Ever heard of cirrhosis of the liver? Maybe, maybe not. In short, it means the hardening of the liver, and it's a serious condition. Apricots can help the liver and its function way before it gets to a condition like cirrhosis. They can help protect against damage to the liver, decrease inflammation and may protect against accrual of fat in the liver. High in beta-carotene, hence the color, they are full of antioxidants that can fight against chronic diseases and prevent cell damage. Apricots reduce inflammation and protect against disease, especially in the large intestines. They're high in fiber, preventing constipation and even hemorrhoids.

Apricots are high in vitamin A, which is good for eye health. Eating one cup of apricots can provide you more than fifty percent of the recommended daily amount. Apricots are an excellent choice whether you eat them raw or dried; if dried, be sure to watch the sugar content.

APPLE CIDER VINEGAR

Most people view vinegar as something to clean with. Others use it to add flavor to their cabbage or other dishes; however, not many think of vinegar with apples. Let me explain. Apple cider vinegar comes from apple cider that has been fermented, making it low in sugar and healthy for you, providing numerous health benefits.

Recently, a new trend started with apple cider vinegar consumption for weight loss. *Is it a fad that will soon fade, or is there something to this?* Actually, ACV helps with weight loss by curbing appetite and breaking down fat accumulation, particularly in the midsection. ACV, in one study, was able to reduce caloric intake up to 275 calories daily.

Do you have acid reflux or gastroesophageal reflux disease (GERD)? ACV reduces acid reflux by adding more acid to the stomach, preventing rear flow, and helps prevent stomach illness.

Did you know taking just two tablespoons a day of apple cider vinegar (diluted, of course) can aid in lowering cholesterol? A study was performed on diabetic and non-diabetic mice, and it measured how ACV affected their lipid profile and total cholesterol. Apple cider vinegar helped the lipids in the normal and diabetic rats while reducing the triglycerides. It also decreased the LDL (bad) cholesterol and increased the HDL (good) cholesterol and may help manage diabetic problems.[5] This does not mean you can still eat high fat foods without getting high cholesterol. A healthy lifestyle and balanced diet while regularly ingesting ACV may help prevent high cholesterol.

Maintaining a balanced blood sugar level is not just important for diabetics but all individuals. ACV helps increase insulin sensitivity, decreases blood sugar levels, and helps them stay balanced, decreasing the frequency of peaks and drops. Also, ACV contains acetic acid, which may help reduce high blood pressure.[6] Now, it is important to balance your sodium, potassium levels, and salt intake, especially

African Americans; however, a case was conducted on hypersensitive rats, and when given ACV, it was observed that vinegar significantly reduced both blood pressure and renin activity compared to controls that were given no acetic acid or vinegar.[7]

Suffering from an upset stomach, maybe an ulcer or even bad internal gut bacteria? Apple cider vinegar can make your gut healthier. It helps digest and absorb foods better, detoxes the body, and makes for healthy gut bacteria.

Acne or scars from previous acne? ACV can improve your skin because of its antibacterial properties, and it kills off acne-causing bacteria. Even if you have hyper-pigmentation or severe scarring, ACV can help decrease the visibility and reduce the amount.[8] Have you experienced warts, fever blisters, or an eye infection? Add ACV to tissue or a cotton swap, and apply it directly to the affected area. Mix ACV with water and drop it into the eye. It will sting initially but help rid any bacteria.

Got a rash or bug bite? ACV contains potassium and can reduce inflammation, swelling, and itchiness. Arthritis is due to inflammation on the joints and can cause intense pain and discomfort. ACV reduces that inflammation, enhances circulation,[9] and eases the pain. ACV is not just for humans; it can be used to kill bugs and fleas on pets. If you're like me, you sweat during an intense workout, but no one wants the odor from a workout to remain on their clothes. ACV is a natural deodorizer. Add some to your detergent, and your clothes will smell clean and fresh. You may even make it into a deodorant for your body; it will neutralize odor.

Lastly, due to the anti-bacterial and anti-fungal properties in apple cider vinegar, it is great for killing fungi. Whether you're dealing with a yeast infection or an open sore, mix ACV with water and use it on the fungus to help eliminate it. Use it on your nails or even your hair. It conditions and detangles hair, removing excess buildup, leaving hair moisturized and shiny.

From topical uses to internal and even for pets, the benefits of apple cider vinegar go on and on. Every household should keep a bottle in the cabinet. Be sure to purchase apple cider vinegar "with the mother."

ALPHA LIPOIC ACID

ALA, or alpha lipoic acid, can help prevent diabetes. It protects cells and nerves in the legs, arms, and other places on the body that are usually associated with diabetes. ALA can lower blood pressure, cholesterol, and even sugar levels.

Ever heard of peripheral neuropathy? It is a "disorder that affects the nerves that provide sensation, which causes pain, tingling, and burning symptoms of the nerves affected."[10] However, ALA can help relieve those symptoms and even reduce swelling and related pain.

Do you have poor vision, maybe cataracts or glaucoma? ALA can help. Several eye diseases are caused by oxidative stress, and ALA can control that stress and decrease or almost stop the oxidative damage in the eye. We all know that as we age, our vision changes, so for those up in age, I highly recommend taking ALA to help prevent vision damage or decline.

ALA is also good for cognitive development and stability. It helps protect memory and can prevent you from having motor impairment. For individuals who are at risk for developing dementia, Alzheimer's, or strokes, ALA can help protect nerve and brain tissue and stimulate cognitive function.

Dealing with skin cancer or skin damage? ALA can help sun lines or even skin damage from the sun. Lastly, ALA helps build your immune system and your glutathione levels.

ALOE VERA

Aloe vera has many benefits, from topical use in the gel form to internal benefits in liquid form. Aloe vera's antimicrobial and antifungal properties can treat herpes, acute dermatitis (also known as eczema), frostbite, acne, and minor inflammation.[11] It helps calm the itching you experience with skin rashes and reduces the amount and frequency of the irritations.

Have you ever wanted to throw down in the kitchen for your spouse, but you burned yourself? What did you do? Next time, grab some aloe as soon as it happens. Aloe helps prevent more damage to the skin, helps new skin cells form faster, and the enzymes it contains reduces pain and inflammation on the affected area, so you can still enjoy that wonderful meal.

Ever get a blister or a cold sore and think, *Man, this itches, and it's an unpleasant sight. How do I get rid of it?* Aloe can help decrease the healing time, and, since it's an anti-inflammatory and fights viral infections, it can decrease your pain and get you back to normal in no time. It also helps with acid reflux and GERD when swallowed, and the B vitamins it contains helps strengthen your immune system to fight off germs in the future.

Dry or itchy scalp? Aloe is a natural moisturizer and can be used on the skin to improve moisture. Its nourishing components can make for a healthy scalp and head of hair. Bad dandruff? Aloe can help you with that, too. It's an antifungal and bacterial plant and therefore rids the head of dead cells and helps restore tissue and follicles.

When ingesting aloe, it's good for constipation, too. Its properties create a laxative that stimulate and increase mucus discharge, therefore helping to break down and mix the food, causing a release. That time of the month and you're bloated? Aloe helps decrease bloating and can even help create a healthy urinary tract.

Aloe helps with digestion and heals stomach ulcers. It balances the stomach acid and PH levels, increases healthy digestive bacteria, and creates a bowel movement. Had a vaginal delivery? Aloe vera is great to help heal and soothe the vagina post baby.

Aloe is packed with vitamins, from zinc that can lower respiratory infections and help children with zinc deficiency, to vitamin A to improve vision and skin. It even has vitamin C, which helps the cardiovascular system, prevents prenatal issues and strengthens immune function. The vitamin E it contains helps protect cells against damage caused by free radicals and works as an antioxidant in the body. Without aloe, you are doing yourself an injustice in more ways than one!

ARTICHOKE

Artichoke is high in vitamins C, A, and K and packed with fiber. It's even great as a dip or with your favorite chicken dish. Artichokes are a versatile yet healthy vegetable. They contain several phytonutrients and antioxidants that help fight against cholesterol, high blood pressure, constipation, and even heart disease. Typically, we consume the artichoke heart, which is the bud of the flower prior to it sprouting.

Artichokes are high in folate and carbohydrates; however, the fiber content is almost just as high as the carbs, making it a great option for low-carb dieters or keto fans. I typically didn't eat artichokes because I wasn't fond of the taste, but once I learned the health benefits, I grew to love them. Packed with antioxidants and vitamin C, artichokes help boost your immune system to fight against infections and illness. They also aid your skin in the production of collagen to promote healthy, firm skin. Our skin is one of our main defenses against infections, and artichokes help strengthen that barrier from the outside in.[12]

I mentioned the fiber that artichokes contain earlier, but let's dive a little deeper. Fiber is huge for humans because it controls how our body processes or breaks down food and determines how our internal readings will come out. Thankfully, for diabetic or pre-diabetic individuals, the artichoke's fibers help balance or normalize blood sugar levels, keeping a steady level throughout instead of highs and lows. It can also help you lose weight. I know you're thinking, *Wait, how?* The fiber helps you feel fuller longer, and artichokes are known to assist in ridding the body of unwanted adipose tissue around the midsection. That means even if you suffer from constipation, upset stomach, diarrhea, or just want to improve your gut flora, artichokes will push the unnecessary toxins and waste, including sugar, out to create a smooth and healthy digestive system.

Are you iron deficient and a vegan or plant-based eater? I am iron deficient, and I always strive to find foods high in iron to avoid taking a supplement because I hate them; that's why I choose artichokes, because they contain about five percent of the daily recommended allowance of iron in just one heart.

Several antioxidants, from quercetin[13] to rutin, are present in artichokes, and these antioxidants protect us from chronic diseases. They combat free radical damage that lead to oxidative stress on the body. One study showed how artichokes may be able to fight against the breast cancer cell line, stating, "AEs (artichokes) reduce cell viability, inhibit cell growth, trigger apoptotic mechanisms, and shows inhibitory properties against the invasive behavior of MDA-MB231 cancer cell line. Altogether, these data indicate the potential chemo-preventive activity of artichoke poly-phenolic extracts."[14]

Another study's findings reported, "Artichoke polyphenols could be a promising dietary tool either in cancer chemoprevention or/and in cancer treatment as a nonconventional, adjuvant therapy."[15] Both studies show the possibility of artichokes helping to prevent cancer.

Do you have high cholesterol, or are you at risk for heart disease? Artichokes assist in lowering cholesterol and combating heart disease due to the soluble fiber inulin, and they reduce chronic inflammation. A study from the National Institute of Health showed artichoke hearts may help fight heart disease due to the "therapeutic properties as the hypolipidemizing[16] activity, antioxidant activity and hypoglycemizing activity."[17]

Raw or cooked, chopped, diced or added to your favorite spinach dip, artichokes are versatile and delicious.

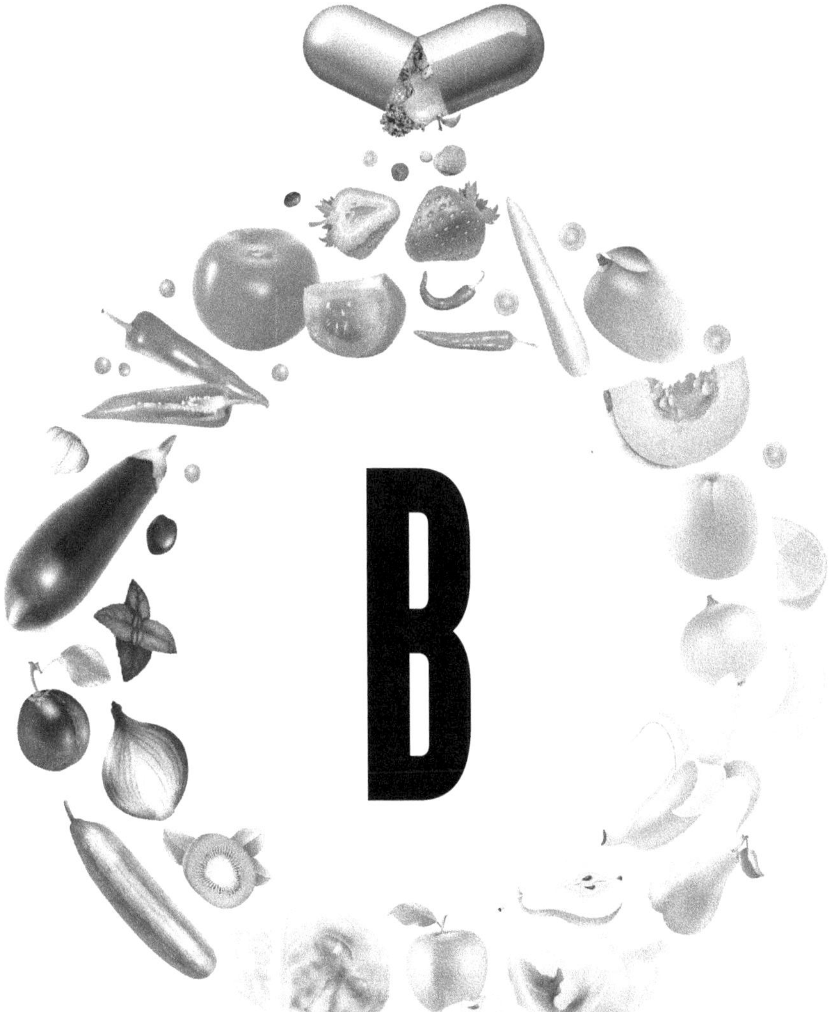
B

BANANAS

Did you know eating one banana can give you up to ninety minutes of non-stop energy? They supply us with carbohydrates that replace the glycogen used during a workout or movement. Now, of course, everyone knows they are high in potassium and can easily provide us with water balance, but what else are they good for? Bananas contain vitamin B6, which regulates our blood sugar levels, and when we're "hangry" or stressed, it can suppress those moods. It's also perfect for us ladies when we're PMS'ing.

Ever eat a banana and feel happy a few minutes after? That's because they release tryptophan, an essential amino acid, which is converted to serotonin, a chemical in the body that heightens your mood and makes you happy.

Are you iron deficient like me? Yeah, I'm sure you're sick of eating spinach, right? Well, bananas are rich in iron and promote production of hemoglobin for us anemic individuals.

Want to pass a test or seem smarter. Eat a banana beforehand. You will be more alert and sharper because bananas help you learn better and remember things.

Tried to quit smoking and failed? Increase your banana intake; they decrease the effects of withdrawal both mentally and physically.

BEETS

Red beets or golden beets—How do you choose? Red beets are high in vitamin C, fiber, and potassium. If you're a heavy drinker or have cirrhosis of the liver, you and beets should be friends. They detoxify the liver and kidneys and are rich in folate, helping to prevent birth defects, which is important for pregnant women.

Beets are high in antioxidants that protect against cancer, and they're high in disease-fighting phytonutrients. They get their deep, rich pigment from betalains, which is an antioxidant that fights illnesses and promotes good eye health. Beets promote a healthy heart because they contain nitrates. They help to improve blood flow and lower blood pressure.

Drinking straight beet juice relieves inflammation and prevents cell damage and oxidative stress. Beets are great for athletes because they provide an instant boost of energy due to the nitrates shown to improve the function of the mitochondria.

Do you deal with diverticulitis or diverticulosis? Beets are high in fiber, aiding in the digestive process and lowering your chances of developing those conditions. Trying to lose weight? Beets are low in calories and will keep you fuller longer because of the high fiber content. The satiation makes you eat less, thus increasing weight loss.

BLUEBERRIES

Often overlooked due to their size, blueberries are considered a superfood, and they're low in calories. From enhancing your memory and promoting good brain health to being high in fiber for a healthy digestive system, blueberries are an antioxidant-filled fruit with lifelong benefits.

These berries contain antioxidants, which are compounds known to fight free radicals. In short, that means they fight against diseases like several cancers, heart disease, and diabetes, just to name a few. Though small, they can reduce your chances of stomach, breast, prostate and different intestinal cancers when consumed regularly with other fruits and vegetables.

Overweight, obese, or just trying to lose a few pounds? Who isn't these days? Blueberries can help; their high fiber content will make you feel and stay fuller longer, decreasing food intake, and one serving contains up to fourteen percent of your recommended daily fiber intake. Stubborn belly fat? Blueberries help decrease stomach fat or adipose tissue in the midsection. Most people don't realize this is the most dangerous area to store fat, but blueberries can help alleviate *a lot* of health problems that develop because of it.

Ever walk into a room and think, *What did I come in here for?* Blueberries are great for short-term memory and cognition. They help promote healthy brain aging, restore memory loss or decline, and protect healthy brain cells.

Now, let's talk about the powerhouse of the body. Yeah, the heart. Blueberries protect your heart in several ways. They help keep your blood pressure low, oxidize LDL's cholesterol, and lower triglycerides. The heart pumps blood throughout the body along with key nutrients, so it's important for it to stay healthy. A healthy heart means lower chances of developing heart disease, high blood pressure (HBP), and even high cholesterol.

Lastly, blueberries fight bladder and urinary tract infections and are good for your skin because they fight against bacteria and promote healthy cell retention.[18] So save yourself and your heart the trouble and eat blueberries while maintaining a healthy lifestyle.

BRUSSELS SPROUTS

Growing up, my mom used to force us to eat Brussels sprouts, and I hated them. She would say, "Honey, they're just baby cabbages, and they're very good for you." I didn't care back then, but now, best believe I always eat Brussels sprouts. Brussels sprouts are part of the cruciferous family, which means they're imperative in fighting cancer. These vegetables fight cancer because they contain sulforaphanes, which inhibit the enzyme involved in progressing cancer cells. Furthermore, we know colon cancer has become more prevalent in today's society, and Brussels sprouts can help reduce the risk because they contain glucosinolates. *What in the world?* All you need to know is these compounds help the body detox itself and increase its defense against pathogens and oxidative stress. They also fight against skin cancer, prostate, pancreatic, esophageal and breast cancer because of the high levels of chlorophyll.

Osteopenia, low bone density, and bone fractures can all be prevented by maintaining healthy bones through sufficient nutrient intake. Vitamin K is responsible for a healthy skeletal system, bone calcification, and decreasing inflammation. Brussels sprouts provide more than 200 percent of the RDA of vitamin K in one serving. Are you vitamin K deficient? If so, these are key on the grocery list for you, and since they're fat soluble, eat them sautéed in avocado oil or with any healthy fat of choice.

The vitamin C in Brussels sprouts helps boost your immune system and reduces inflammation and cell damage. The antioxidants keep your immune system strong against bacteria, viruses, and harmful invaders that can cause disease and illness. Brussels sprouts can prevent autoimmune diseases like rheumatoid arthritis because they protect cells from free radical damage and help maintain a healthy digestive tract system, a healthy mouth, and integumentary system.

Studies have shown that chronic inflammation is correlated with several diseases and disorders, so decreasing inflammation will help prevent heart disease, cognitive disorders, and even diabetes.

Brussels sprouts contain vitamin K, vitamin C, antioxidants, and omega-3 fatty acids, which clean the arteries of unwanted plaque and increase blood flow for healthy blood vessels and low blood pressure.

When I mentioned that Brussels sprouts are good for digestive health, I was not only referring to constipation and getting in enough fiber. The glucosinolates present in Brussels sprouts are metabolites that fight against pathogens, according to sciencedirect.com, and they help protect the lining of the stomach and intestines, helping to prevent leaky gut syndrome. Brussels sprouts also detoxify the body by riding it of unwanted waste and bacteria, causing a decrease in blood pressure and cholesterol due to the high fiber content.

Work outside in the sun? Always looking for thicker sunglasses or a higher SPF sunscreen? Eating Brussels sprouts can help because of the vitamin C they contain, helping to protect the skin from UV damage and slowing down the skin aging process. Also, vitamin A protects the eyes from harmful light rays and reduces oxidative stress, which could lead to cataracts and macular degeneration.

Are you at risk for developing diabetes? Already pre-diabetic or have a family history of diabetes? I do. Brussels sprouts can help prevent you from developing diabetes because it increases your insulin sensitivity and decreases inflammation. If you already have diabetes, it can lower your glucose levels and reduce further diabetic complications.

Brussels sprouts are full of folate, which is necessary for a healthy baby and delivery. They're also high in potassium for essential nerve function, metabolizing carbs, and muscle contraction.

So I guess the old saying stays true: "Mom knows best!"

BROCCOLI

Broccoli is one of my favorite vegetables to eat. When I was a child, I *loved* them because they reminded me of small trees.

Broccoli is one of the main vegetables to eat to help fight cancer because it targets carcinogens, helping to stop damage from reoccurring and affecting the DNA and healthy cells. It also fights against toxins found in the body. With cervical cancer becoming more prevalent, all individuals, especially women, must pay attention and eat more broccoli because it may help increase good estrogen and reduce chances of developing certain cancers.

Broccoli aids in weight loss because it is considered a complex carbohydrate, meaning you won't be hungry one hour later, and it is slowly digested, creating prolonged satiation. It promotes healthy skin because of its vitamin C, which helps repair the damage caused from skin products or the sun. It even protects the eyes due to its vitamin A properties and carotenoids, which keep eyes healthy as we age and decreases vision disorders. Want to detox your body or go on a cleanse? No need; just eat some broccoli. It naturally cleanses your blood and digestive system due to its compounds and high fiber. It will increase your healthy gut flora and immunity and rid your body of unwanted bacteria all at the same time.

Broccoli is good for your heart because it helps bind cholesterol and removes it from the body before even entering the blood stream, thus giving you a lower chance for cardiovascular disease. It helps fight against free radical damage and is high in calcium. The high calcium is good for building and maintaining strong bones and teeth. A lot of Americans are calcium and iron deficient, and broccoli contains both.

From vitamin K to help with bone density to magnesium and iron to maintain healthy nails, broccoli is way more than just a small green tree! Just remember one thing: Eating broccoli causes a lot of gas because it's a cruciferous vegetable, so avoid going on a first date after eating it.

BEAN SPROUTS

Ever heard of them? They are those long, white sprouts usually found at a salad bar. *But what do they do?*

Well, for one, they contain manganese, which is one of the key nutrients needed to keep strong bones. The older we get, the weaker our bones become unless we intake the nutrients needed to maintain their strength. We all know that iron is found in broccoli and spinach, but did you know bean sprouts contain iron, too? Yes, the iron found in bean sprouts can help us stay infection free and maintain optimal health by killing off unwanted germs and pathogens.

While we're on the topic of iron, let's focus on blood. Some people suffer from prolonged bleeding and blood clot failure. Bean sprouts are full of vitamin K, which is needed in the blood clotting process and can even help reduce the risk of heart disease, according to *Medical News Today*.

Lastly, bean sprouts can make you smile. They contain vitamin C, which may reduce your stress levels and anxiety. It can even help you stay calm in difficult or stressful situations. So the next time you have a big project at work that is going to cause anxiety, eat some bean sprouts ahead of time!

BLACK SEED OIL

Is it an oil or a seed? Well, it's an oil that comes from a seed. Its primary health benefit is that it reduces excess growth of yeast in the body due to its antifungal properties.[19]

Black seed oil comes from black cumin seeds called nigella sativa. It also helps with rheumatoid arthritis, asthma, high blood pressure, high cholesterol, and even an upset stomach. And black seed oil combats many more illnesses due to the phytochemicals it contains. The primary three phytochemicals that contribute to black seed oil's benefits are thymol, thymoquinone, and thymohydroquinone, enabling black seed oil to fight off chronic diseases such as cancer. One research study found that black seed oil was able to "inhibit development of pancreatic cancer as a result of its anti-inflammatory properties. Also, the herb inhibited the activation and synthesis of NF-kappaB, a transcription factor that has been implicated in inflammation-associated cancer. Activation of NF-kappaB has been observed in pancreatic cancer and may be a factor in pancreatic cancer's resistance to chemotherapeutic agents."[20]

Black seed oil helps reduce inflammation and inhibits immune disorders. Both thymoquinone and thymohydroquinone showed anti-tumor effects when given to trial mice.[21]

Have you ever used a special hand cream for dry, cracked skin, eczema, and frequent washing (like in a hospital)? Black seed oil may be more effective at keeping the skin moisturized and preventing eczema. One study showed that Nigella sativa might have the same efficacy as betamethasone in improvement of life quality and decreasing the severity of hand eczema.[22]

Have you recently taken a lot of medication, or were you previously a heavy drinker? Often, we can cause damage to our liver without being aware of the severity. Black seed oil may help improve liver function and reduce further damage.

Sugar is one of the main problems for people today because it is found in everything, and we can easily become addicted to it. Excessive sugar intake leads to diabetes, unwanted weight gain, unnecessary toxins in the body, and chronic diseases.

However, black seed oil may help improve and prevent diabetes. "N. sativa (black seed) can help diabetic individuals and those with glucose intolerance because it helps reduce appetite, glucose absorption in intestine, hepatic gluconeogenesis, blood glucose level, cholesterol, triglycerides, body weight, and it stimulates insulin from beta-cells in the pancreas; improves glucose tolerance as efficiently as metformin; yet it has not shown any side effects and has low toxicity."[23]

Many women want long, luscious hair, but some of us struggle to achieve it. I have a dry scalp, so I always have dandruff. Others have severe shedding or alopecia. Black seed oil helps moisturize the hair, and due to its antifungal, antibacterial, and antiviral properties and its antihistamines, it heals and improves scalp health while helping to re-grow and repair hair follicles.[24]

Since we've already focused on the ladies for hair growth, now, men, it's your turn. Struggle with fertility or low sperm count? Black seed oil may improve sperm count and improve fertility. One study conducted of men who were infertile or had a sperm count less than thirty percent showed a "daily intake of 5ml N. sativa oil for two months improves abnormal semen quality in infertile men without any adverse effects."[25]

Have you ever heard of MSRA or methicillin-resistant staphylococcus aureus? It is an antibiotic-resistant infection, and it's mostly found in hospitals for the elderly or those with weak immune systems due to multiple surgeries. Why am I telling you this? Black seed oil may stop or decrease the rate at which the infection will spread.

One study states, "Results indicated that N. sativa has an inhibitory effect on MRSA."[26]

Finally, hypertension or high blood pressure are common diagnoses, especially for minorities, and we are always looking for ways to lower our numbers. One study was conducted on individuals who had mild hypertension and the effect taking black seed oil had on them. The results suggested, "The daily use of NS seed extract for two months may have a blood-pressure-lowering effect in patients with mild HT."[27]

Black seed oil may also help improve hypertension and help with overall heart health and function. From the hair to the skin, fertility and infections, black seed oil is a powerhouse and should be—no, needs to be—in your home!

BERBERINE

This natural extract is found in Chinese and Indian medicine and can be used as a natural antibiotic to treat conditions instead of resorting to pharmaceutical drugs. Berberine has many antimicrobial, antifungal, and anti-inflammatory properties that can significantly help with overall health and wellness.

Do you have diabetes or diabetic neuropathy? Berberine has been shown to lower blood glucose levels and "improve insulin sensitivity by adjusting adipokine secretion."[28]

Furthermore, it can lower cholesterol by decreasing fats and lipids in the bloodstream and getting rid of the cholesterol in the liver, preventing its absorption in the intestines. Berberine can also help lower your triglyceride levels, and when combined with red yeast rice, according to a study in *Metabolism*, "has a bigger range of overall cholesterol protection than that of satin[29] drugs."[30]

Berberine can also help fight against obesity by activating an enzyme in the body known to regulate metabolism. Once the enzyme is activated, it boosts fat burning in the mitochondria. This, in turn, decreases fat buildup in the body.

Berberine also helps the heart. We previously discussed the positive effects it has on obesity and blood pressure, which coincides with heart disease. Berberine lowers the risk for heart disease. It protects against clogged arteries or atherosclerosis due to the release of a molecule that relaxes the arteries and increases blood flow.

Are you a smoker or were you a smoker in your past life? Since we know berberine to be an anti-inflammatory, it promotes healthy lungs by decreasing inflammation of the alveoli caused by smoking. So next time you're in your favorite supermarket, stop by the vitamin section and pick up some berberine.

BROCCOLI SPROUTS

Not to be confused as mini-broccoli, broccoli sprouts are the forerunner to traditional broccoli. They are often overlooked or thought of as having little to no nutritional benefit because of their small size; however, they're packed with benefits and are one of the top cancer-fighting foods. Broccoli sprouts contain an enzyme called myrosinase,[31] which works with healthy gut bacteria to break down glucosinolates into a functional form to fight against disease. To receive these benefits, try to eat the broccoli sprouts in raw form, easily added to a salad. These sprouts contain big amounts of glucoraphanin, the glucosinolate precursor to the isothiocyanate sulforaphane. This knowledge is important because broccoli sprouts may be able to reduce inflammation and further harm to someone who has suffered a brain injury. According to one study, "Post-injury administration of sulforaphane (SUL), an isothiocyanate present in abundance in cruciferous vegetables such as broccoli, decreased AQP4 (water) loss in the injury core and further increased AQP4 levels in the brain. These increases in AQP4 levels were accompanied by a significant reduction in brain edema (assessed by percentage water content) at three days post-injury."[32]

Daily, we take toxins into our bodies, from the foods we eat to the air we breathe. A study was performed in an area with a lot of airborne pollutants that typically cause respiratory issues and asthma. The study was to measure the amount of toxins excreted through urine with the supplementation of sulforaphane and without. The results indicated a higher excretion of toxins in the subjects that had sulforaphane than those without. Thus, intervention with broccoli sprouts enhances the detoxification of some airborne pollutants and may provide a frugal means to attenuate their associated long-term health risks.[33]

This enzyme may help rid the body of unnecessary toxins and

improve respiratory function. One of the main causes of asthma is chronic inflammation and restricted airways, and pollutants increase airway restriction and cause oxidative stress.[34] Sulforaphane may also be able to lessen the effect of toxins in respiratory epithelial cells and show chemo-preventive potential.

Have you ever heard of H. pylori, or do you know someone who has experienced it? It is an infection or pathogen that causes inflammation and damage in the stomach. However, studies show that broccoli sprouts may protect the gastric lining of the stomach and reduce associated inflammation to combat the infection.[35]

Lastly, but more importantly, broccoli sprouts may be able to inhibit and help combat cancer.[36] Recent identification of a sub-population of tumor cells with a stem cell-like self-renewal capacity that may be responsible for relapse, metastasis, and resistance, as a potential target of the dietary compound, may be an important aspect of sulforaphane chemoprevention. Evidence also suggests that sulforaphane may target the epigenetic alterations observed in specific cancers, reversing aberrant changes in gene transcription through mechanisms of histone deacetylase inhibition, global demethylation, and microRNA modulation.[37] That means that sulforaphane may be able to stop cancer cells from spreading, reverse damage, and detoxify carcinogens in the body. More research is being conducted daily on which types of cancer and the level of severity in prevention.

Though they are small, they are mighty. Don't overlook broccoli sprouts because you could save yourself serious disease development in the future.

BLACK ELDERBERRY

Is black elderberry a berry just like strawberries and blueberries?
Not quite, elderberry comes from the elder plant, native to Europe
and Africa. It's used as a medicinal herb for its antiviral effects, and
when taken at the first signs of infections or cold symptoms, it can
help shorten the duration of the illness. Elderberries contain flavonoids
and compounds such as quercetin and rutin, also anthocyanins and
antioxidants, all which help fight against cell damage and boost the
immune system.[38] Typically, elderberry comes in liquid form, but it
also can be consumed in a vitamin or even a tea if you purchase the
berries dried.

Now that we have a little background on the elderberry, let's dig into
how it can benefit us. Elderberries may be able to improve heart health,
from cholesterol to blood pressure. The berry contains anthocyanins,[39]
which are polyphenols that have demonstrated antioxidant and anti-
inflammatory properties. One study was performed on mice to determine
if the elderberry was able to protect against chronic inflammation
and atherosclerosis (hardening of the arteries). The results indicated
"significant reductions in total cholesterol content of the aorta of black
elderberry fed mice, indicating less atherosclerosis progression. This
study suggests that black elderberry may have the potential to influence
HDL dysfunction associated with chronic inflammation by impacting
hepatic gene expression."[40]

On the other hand, I previously mentioned infections and colds
and how elderberry may be able to decrease the amount of time you're
ill if taken at the onset of the symptoms, but you may be wondering
how. The anthocyanins combat damage to the cells and stimulate the
immune system, while the anti-microbial effect helps fight against
bacterial infections. Research has shown elderberry to be effective in
fighting against the flu, herpes, and influenza.[41]

Also, if you suffer from allergies and constant sneezing, one way the immune system responds to irritation and inflammation in the nasal cavity, elderberries' anthocyanins help improve the symptoms and decrease the frequency of a reaction. One study showed the effect elderberry had on people's wellbeing after traveling across the world and how their cold symptoms were affected after taking the berry. The results showed "a significant reduction of cold duration and severity."[42]

Ever experienced sinusitis or a sinus infection? I have, and they are *painful*! Well, we know elderberry is an antiviral and anti-inflammatory, so there's no doubt it is a great herb to use in helping to ease the pain and relieve a sinus infection.[43]

Do you have edema, or are you pregnant and retaining unnecessary water? Elderberry is a great natural diuretic, which can help relieve the unwanted swelling, water, and pain you experience and remove toxins from the digestive system. Cancer is, sadly, a widely common disease, and we are always looking for prevention or ways to fight against cancer. One study showed elderberry in the native form from Europe (Sambucus nigra) and the American form (Sambucus canadensis) may have cancer fighting properties. "Both cultivated S. nigra and wild S. canadensis fruits demonstrated significant chemo-preventive potential through strong induction of quinone reductase and inhibition of cyclooxygenase-2, which is indicative of anti-initiation and anti-promotion properties, respectively. In addition, fractions of S. canadensis extract showed inhibition of ornithine decarboxylase, an enzyme marker related to the promotion stage of carcinogenesis."[44]

Elderberry is also helpful for high blood sugar. Yes, diabetics, elderberry has something to help you. It has insulin-releasing and insulin-like activity and may lower blood sugar levels naturally. In a recent study, elderberry "significantly increased 2-deoxy-glucose transport, glucose oxidation and glycogenesis (where sugar is moved out of the bloodstream and into the muscles) of mouse abdominal muscle in the absence of added insulin."[45]

Elderberry is high in vitamins C and A, iron, and much more to protect our bodies from toxins, oxidative stress, and damage. Don't think of it as just another berry; think of elderberry as medicine to heal yourself naturally from the inside out.[46]

BLACKBERRIES

Blackberries are one of the best fruits to eat. They are known for their cancer-fighting properties. They contain anthocyanins, which are phytochemicals, and according to The National Library of Medicine, they are the number one way to fight against development of cancer and cell mutation. Blackberries also contain vitamin K, which is known to help prevent oral, stomach, liver, nasal, colon, and prostate cancers.

Blackberries are also great for brain health since they contain manganese, which is vital for adequate brain function. Do you have epilepsy or frequent seizures? Blackberries can help. They help prevent brain degeneration and keep the synapses of the brain firing. With inflammation being the root cause of so many diseases we see today, foods like blackberries that fight inflammation are underutilized and underappreciated. Blackberries reduce inflammation and allow the body's systems to more easily function naturally. From protecting the body against stomach ulcers, oxidative stress, inflammation, and bloating from menstruation, blackberries should be considered a superfood.

Thought we were finished? Oh, no! Blackberries are also good for the cardiovascular system and even the skin. The vitamin K they contain also stops the hardening of arteries and prevents plaque buildup, which keeps a healthy blood pressure. Furthermore, blackberries keep you looking good by protecting the skin from UV damage and promoting collagen production. The antiviral effect they have relieves cold sores and other infections prone to the skin.

If you have diverticulitis or diverticulosis, stay away from this berry. The small bubbles you see are drupelets and could get stuck in your digestive system.

BIOTIN

Do you want healthy nails and long, luscious hair? Biotin is the key! Several women and men suffer from cracked, brittle, dry hair and nails, but little do they know biotin can help resolve that issue. It can be found primarily in eggs. But biotin has other health benefits besides promoting strong nails and hair. Biotin, or vitamin B7, supports a healthy metabolism by means of converting the food and sugars or glucose we eat into usable energy. Biotin also helps diabetics because it assists insulin activity and decreases the properties that stimulate glucose, so less sugar goes into the bloodstream, keeping the sugar levels balanced and low. B vitamins like biotin are good for cognitive development and brain function. They regulate and synthesize hormones, especially ones that affect your cognition and mood. They also help decrease your chances of developing dementia and Alzheimer's, diseases related to brain and cognitive function.

Trouble losing weight or thyroid issues? Biotin helps fight adrenal fatigue and supports a healthy thyroid. The adrenal and thyroid glands affect everything from your mood to your energy level and even your sleep patterns; therefore, they should be balanced and regulated at all times.

Workout a lot and always sore after? Biotin helps repair muscles and makes them grow stronger and at a faster rate. When it comes to muscle tissues and fibers, biotin repairs the tiny tears made when working out to decrease inflammation and aid in proper development.

So now you can have it all—healthy hair, nails, and a fit body!

BANANA PEPPERS

There are green peppers, yellow, spicy, or mild. How do we know which to pick? Banana peppers are a great choice. That's right, not bananas and not the traditional pepper, but banana peppers. *Are they hot or spicy?* No, banana peppers are five times milder than traditional peppers and provide an enormous amount of health benefits. Just like jalapeno peppers, banana peppers contain capsaicin, a compound that makes things spicy, but these are not hot at all. For men especially, capsaicin is important because it is known to help kill prostate cancer cells. Also, it can prevent sinus infections, and its antibacterial properties help fight symptoms related to infections, according to yourhealthremedy.com.

A great thing about banana peppers is they are full of vitamin C and folate, which are good for maintaining a healthy heart and immune system. The vitamin C helps reduce gout, a complex form of inflammatory arthritis when too much uric acid is present, and the vitamin B6 they contain helps control the aches and pains present in individuals with arthritis. Vitamin C is beneficial because it is needed to make collagen, which is used in our bones, cartilage, and tendons of the body.

Banana peppers decrease your risk of heart disease because B6 and folate combined reduce homocysteine levels, which come from amino acid in the blood and keep your cholesterol and blood pressure levels stable.

Finally, these peppers help eliminate free radical damage and help maintain healthy brain function.

BOK CHOY

Often used in the Asian culture or in stir-fry, bok choy is a form of cabbage and is one of the most nutrient-dense foods you can eat. It is considered a cruciferous vegetable, meaning it is full of vitamin K, folate, and phytonutrients that help fight cancer and other chronic diseases.[47] It's packed with antioxidants that fight free radial damage and help reduce chronic inflammation, the main cause of disease today. Bok choy contains more vitamin A and vitamin C in one serving than our recommended daily allowance.[48]

Also, if you're aiming to lose weight for an event or just drop a few pounds, bok choy helps detoxify the body and rids it of excess waste. Since it's low in calories but high in fiber, it will keep you fuller longer, aiding in decreased appetite.

Cabbage contains phenols and compounds that the body uses to combat pathogens and invaders to maintain a healthy system. Bok choy's polyphenols may help improve high cholesterol and have a direct positive affect on cell membranes. One study on the affect cruciferous vegetables has on cancer prevention[49] states the results "clearly point toward a positive correlation between cancer prevention of many target organs and consumption of cruciferous vegetables or their active constituents."[50]

Bok choy contains an antimicrobial called brassinin, which research suggests may have chemo-preventive properties and the ability to inhibit cancer cells.[51]

Are you elderly or calcium deficient? Has your physician explained that you may be at risk for developing osteoporosis? Bok choy contains calcium, phosphorus, vitamin K, and iron, which all work together to maintain good bone health. If you're like me and vitamin D deficient, bok choy contains vitamin D to help with bone density and the growth of healthy bones. One study from the National Institute of Health reported, "There is a consistent line of evidence in human epidemiologic and intervention studies that clearly demonstrates that vitamin K can improve bone health. The human intervention studies have demonstrated that vitamin K can not only increase bone mineral density in osteoporotic people but also actually reduce fracture rates. Further, there is evidence in human intervention studies that vitamins K and D, classics in bone metabolism, work synergistically on bone density."[52]

Are you thinking about expanding your family? No, I am not talking about purchasing a pet, but having a baby. It is important for the mother to take in key nutrients prior to conception, during pregnancy, and after the baby is born. Folate is one of the key nutrients needed for proper cell development and helps fight against spinal bifida and neural tube defects. Folate[53] is necessary for the production of the baby's blood cells and spinal cord.

Do you have bad acne, eczema, or hair loss? Bok choy contains high amounts of vitamin C, which helps produce collagen. Collagen aids in maintaining firm, tight skin, reducing wrinkles, and it helps with hair production, growth, and revitalization. The antibacterial and antioxidant compounds fight against inflammation in the skin and infections such as severe acne or eczema.

We know vitamin C is good for our immune system when we're sick, fighting infections and illness, and strengthening it to prevent further illness; however, bok choy also contains the mineral selenium. Often overlooked, it aids in the development of our helper T-cells, which are key in combating illness.

Do you have high blood pressure? A lot of African Americans do because of poor diet choices, and we're already at risk due to our ancestry. When I learned this, I researched foods that could naturally help prevent high blood pressure and improve my heart health. Potassium is one of the key nutrients that can naturally help lower blood pressure while balancing sodium levels. "Epidemiological and clinical studies show that a high-potassium diet lowers blood pressure in individuals with both raised blood pressure and average population blood pressure. Prospective cohort studies and outcome trials show that increasing potassium intake reduces cardiovascular disease mortality. This is mainly attributable to the blood-pressure-lowering effect and may also be partially because of the direct effects of potassium on the cardiovascular system."[54]

Earlier, I mentioned the high amount of vitamin A in bok choy, but let me explain why that is necessary. One of the first ways we remember things is by what we see. We retain the information and play it over in our brains. Vitamin A, along with beta-carotene, helps protect our eyes from free radical damage and even helps block the UV rays from the sun to prevent damage. Macular degeneration is a disease that can often lead to blurry vision and even blindness; however, vitamin A combats the effects and treats dry eyes to improve overall eye health. Bok choy may even help reduce your risk of developing cataracts.[55]

It is important to take preventive measures before you are diagnosed to help live a long, healthy lifestyle.

You can eat bok choy raw or cooked, and it is best harvested in the winter due to its delicate leaves, so try it in one of your favorite soups.

BRAZIL NUTS

Brazil nuts are a fat. *What? Fats are bad!* No, no, it's a mono-unsaturated fat, meaning it's a "good fat." *Whew!* Also, it is high in protein for my vegans and one of the highest selenium-rich foods. Selenium helps fight cancer and improve thyroid function by regulating oxygen within the thyroid, decreasing your chance of developing thyroid disease. Brazil nuts also contain ellagic, which is an antioxidant that protects against neurological damage.[56]

They can also improve your serotonin levels, which will heighten your mood, make you happy, and decrease feelings of anxiety. From improving high cholesterol to depression, cancer and even stroke, Brazil nuts provide numerous benefits. Just don't eat more than two or three, especially while taking a multivitamin with selenium because it can lead to selenium toxicity.

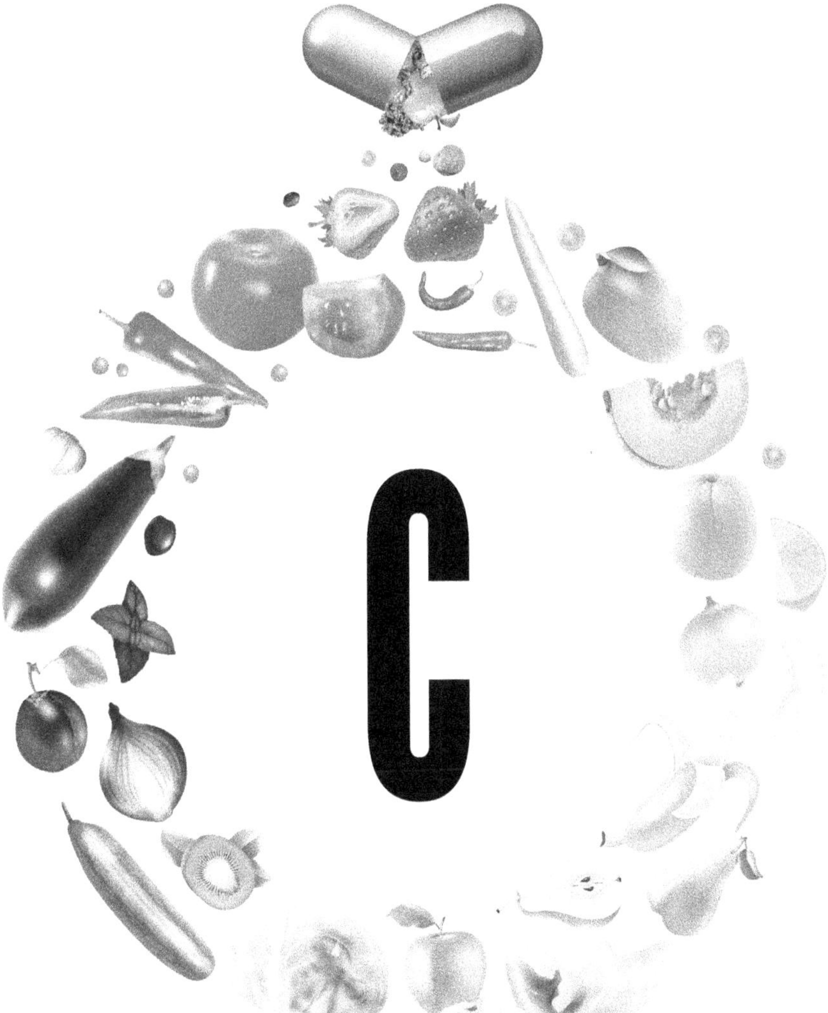
C

COFFEE

It's the thing that millions of Americans must have every morning to be productive citizens. There's always a line at the coffee shop, and it sometimes costs four to six dollars for a small cup. Coffee gets such a bad rep, and people claim it's not healthy, but let's be honest ... Actually, coffee bean is excellent for you and has great health benefits; it's the added cream and sugar that's not so healthy. Coffee can help decrease your chances of developing type 2 diabetes, dementia, heart arrythmias, or stroke. It helps fight constipation, Parkinson's disease, and Alzheimer's. Coffee is full of antioxidants, which help fight free radicals and aid in protecting us from the thousands of toxins we encounter daily. It also contains minerals that help the body use insulin and regulate blood sugar.

"For Parkinson's disease, the data have always been very consistent: Higher consumption of coffee is associated with decreased risk of Parkinson's," Hu tells WebMD.[57]

Coffee helps with Alzheimer's because it improves mental ability and cognitive function by increasing blood flow to the brain.

Coffee is also a natural diuretic, which means if you frequently suffer from constipation or just need a good cleansing, drink coffee, and I promise you will soon feel better.

Lastly, we all know coffee makes you more alert and energized, hence why we drink it in the morning to get us going for the day, but did you know that same effect can work with physical activity? According to draxe.com, "A 2009 study published in *Sports Medicine* shows that coffee increases alertness and improves mental and physical performance in the short run."[58]

So the next time you think about skipping out on that cup of Joe, don't. Grab it and enjoy it; just make sure you watch your intake of all the additives.

CARROTS

You can boil them, eat them raw, even juice them. Rabbits love them, kids enjoy them, and parents will tolerate them. Carrots are known for their rich color. They get their deep, rich orange color from carotenes, which are antioxidants, and one in particular is beta-carotene. If you have ever received an eye exam, then you know carrots are great for vision and eye health. Carrots are full of vitamins C, K, and, most importantly, vitamin A. Just one cup of carrots contains more than triple the RDA of Vitamin A. Vitamin A is directly linked to our vision and vitamin A deficiency can lead to macular degeneration or even blindness.[59] The antioxidants also help fight viruses and inflammation, protect cells from damage, and fight free radicals.

We have to protect our hearts, especially as women, because we bare children and our bodies must be able to handle the stress that comes along with it. Carrots help decrease chances of heart disease and stroke by lowering cholesterol and helping the body digest adipose tissue or fat. Furthermore, it decreases oxidative stress and strengthens your body's defense to fight off harmful pathogens.

So we talked about the benefits carrots have on the heart, but what about the brain? Carrots help improve brain function and decrease inflammation or stress on the brain.[60] Also, they can "weaken nerve signaling, thus protecting against Alzheimer's disease and memory loss."[61]

Lastly, carrots have antibacterial minerals that can fight bacteria in the body by "scrubbing" the digestive system with its high fiber content. It even does scrubbing literally in the mouth by removing unwanted plaque, buildup, and toxins that live in the mouth. The high fiber content helps fight infection and can aid in healing topical scrapes and cuts. Whether you choose to eat carrots or juice them and drink it, try your best to keep them in your diet.

CHIA SEEDS

They are a superfood and sometimes added to drinks or even made into a pudding. Did you know "chia" means strength in the Mayan language? No, well the name alone should tell you it has a lot of strong health benefits for us. Chia seeds are full of fiber, vitamins and minerals, antioxidants, and even healthy fats. From cancer, to weight loss, diabetes and digestive health, and much more, chia seeds can help.

Are you at a higher risk of developing cervical or breast cancer? Maybe your doctor has informed you or it runs in your family history. Chia seeds can help! They are known as cancer-fighting seeds, and due to their richness of ALA, or alpha lipoic acid, they can help fight cancer cells without damaging healthy cells. "The *Journal of Molecular Biochemistry* found that ALA limited the growth of cancer cells in both breast and cervical cancers."[62]

Chia seeds can also help develop and maintain strong bones. They contain boron, which is essential for bone health and has more than fifteen percent of the RDA of calcium. Strong bones include your teeth, and chia seeds help with overall mouth health by preventing plaque buildup on the teeth because they contain zinc.

What about their high fiber content, how does that benefit us? Chia seeds are imperative for digestive health. The high fiber keeps you fuller longer, which aids in weight loss. Also, the fiber helps keep you regular with frequent bowel movements and balances out blood sugar levels, thus helping prevent type 2 diabetes.[63]

Ever put a chia seed in your mouth and just let it sit there without swallowing it? It formed a jelly-like texture, right? Chia seeds form that jelly texture because they are a soluble fiber and a prebiotic, aiding in overall gut health. One interesting thing about chia seeds is that they can expand up to triple their size in water, thus improving adsorption of nutrients and prolonging hydration.

On the other hand, they are a great source of protein, especially for my vegans who have plant-based diets. They can help boost your metabolism, and since they're high in zinc, they will help increase your endurance and stamina during exercise.

Earlier, we talked about how chia seeds help with blood sugar, but they can also help halt and reverse diabetes. These little seeds are packed with omega-3 fatty acids and help lower blood pressure, balance cholesterol, and decrease chances of developing atherosclerosis or hardening of the arteries because they can reverse oxidative stress and decrease inflammation.

Chia seeds' ability to help you maintain a healthy heart and overall healthy body is phenomenal and reminds us why the name means strength.

CANTALOUPE

Did you know your body actually sees this fruit as a vegetable? *What?* Crazy, right? Cantaloupes are orange in color because they're filled with beta-carotene. *Isn't that what carrots have?* Yes! Beta-carotene is also in carrots, and it is a carotenoid that gives fruits and vegetables their color. Cantaloupe is filled with vitamin C, which we know helps maintain strong bones and cartilage due to its activity in the production of collagen. Furthermore, cantaloupes help with the common cold and prevalent diseases such as cancer and diabetes. The antioxidants present in cantaloupes have been shown to protect cells against damage and fight free radicals. Also, "Studies show that cantaloupe's antioxidants and cucurbitacins result in cancerous cell apoptosis, or self-destruction of the cancerous cells. These helpful chemical pheromones exist naturally in plants to protect the plants from external damage, but they also do the same within the human body"[64].

When it's the middle of the summer and it's scorching hot outside, what do you do? Grab some cantaloupe. They're filled with water and help maintain proper hydration. Also, they contribute to a healthy heart because when you're properly hydrated, your heart doesn't have to work as hard to pump blood throughout the body.

Cantaloupe is also good for your liver and kidneys because they detoxify the body and support proper digestion.

Pregnant or thinking about becoming pregnant? Cantaloupe is filled with folic acid, which is known to decrease a baby's chances of developing neural tube defects and improve overall baby health while in the womb.

Do you workout a lot? Ever caught a cramp out of nowhere and didn't know why? Potassium. It is important that your body gets enough potassium. Cantaloupe provides about fourteen percent of the

RDA of potassium and helps keep the right potassium balance to have great nerve function and muscle contractions.

Cantaloupe is also an alkaline food, meaning it can help restore your body to its natural pH levels, thus decreasing the chance of disease formation.

All this information about cantaloupe is great, but I don't know how to pick one. Here's a little pro tip: You should be able to smell the cantaloupe and its ripeness when you pick it up. The aroma should be sweet and pleasant, and the outside texture should be firm and a little heavy. Then you know you've got a good one!

CELERY

How do you eat it, with peanut butter, hummus? I love it in soups and raw for a snack. Most of us have eaten celery in some form or another, and it is excellent for you! It helps with cancer, lung health, weight loss, ulcers, blood pressure, and the list goes on. But let's examine just a few of the health benefits. Celery can help fight against cancer, especially breast cancer, because it contains polyacetylenes. Polyacetylenes are compounds that have been shown to be "highly toxic towards fungi, bacteria, and mammalian cells and display neurotoxic, anti-inflammatory, and anti-platelet-aggregatory effects. Also, the effects of these polyacetylenes toward human cancer cells, their human bioavailability, and their ability to reduce tumor formation in a mammalian in vivo model indicates that they may also provide benefits for health."[65]

In essence, celery can help fight cancer and reduce the formation of tumors.

Have frequent UTIs or urinary tract infections? Celery can help you because it's known for its anti-microbial properties that fight off bacterial infections and increase urination while decreasing uric acid, which is beneficial for getting rid of a UTI.

Ever eat a bunch of celery with peanut butter and notice your stomach starts hurting, and you have to use the restroom? I know, me too. It's because celery is a natural diuretic and is filled with water. Therefore, it reduces bloating and decreases water retention all while improving gut circulation and causing a bowel movement.

Trying to lose weight? Celery is very low in calories and full of nutrients. It will not only boost your metabolism but also control how your fat is metabolized. The lipid or fat metabolism is great for the liver as well because it helps prevent fat buildup in and around the liver, helping to maintain a healthy organ.

Is high blood pressure a common disease in your family? Most African Americans are prone to high blood pressure. However, celery can help prevent and even treat high blood pressure. Celery seeds contain anti-hypertensive properties. That means celery can "help lower high blood pressure by acting as a smooth muscle relaxant and also improves the flow of calcium and potassium into and out of cells. Celery extract helps blood vessels expand and contract, improve blood flow, and aid in overall heart health."[66]

Celery can also lower your cholesterol by helping reduce lipid or fat in the heart as mentioned earlier. It's an anti-inflammatory and fights against chronic inflammation, which is the cause of most major diseases.

So whether you eat it raw, jazz it up with some hummus, or create a kids' snack like ants on a log (raisins and peanut butter on a celery stick), make sure you add this nutrient-dense, disease-fighting food to your daily routine.

CHERRIES

As a kid, I always looked forward to summer because I knew we could find some ripe and juicy cherries. You know the saying, "The darker the berry, the sweeter the juice." This applies to cherries, too. Cherries help to keep the vagina, or "berry," clean when eaten regularly, and they're sweet. Deep red cherries provide more nutrients than rainier cherries. Cherries are typically known, by women anyway, to fight urinary tract infections, but they are great for weight loss, cancer prevention, inflammation, gout, and they even aid in getting proper rest; let's see how.

"A research study was done at the University of Michigan, and it showed that tart cherries activate PPAR isoforms (peroxisome proliferator activating receptors) in many of the body's tissues. PPARs regulate genes that are involved in fat and glucose metabolism, and when modified, they can help reduce the risk of cardiovascular disease."[67]

Also, cherries are high in antioxidants, which aids in fighting against inflammation, cell damage, heart disease, and cancer. Furthermore, cherries fight against free radicals and contain vitamin A, which prevents macular degeneration and glaucoma and promotes healthy skin.[68]

Cherries can even help with the pain of gout. *What is gout?* Gout is an arthritic condition due to the excess buildup of uric acid in the body. Cherries can help reduce inflammation in the lower body and reduce uric acid levels typically caused by gout. Trouble sleeping at night or staying asleep? You may have heard that melatonin can aid in sleeping, but did you know cherries contain phytochemicals like melatonin, which can help you sleep better? It's true. I mentioned previously that cherries are great for weight loss, but how? Cherries help decrease the production of fat in the blood and are great for bowel movements which, in turn, keeps weight down. So just remember, the darker the berry the sweeter the juice, literally!

CAT'S CLAW

Cat's claw is a plant or an herb used to treat lots of different symptoms and diseases. It can treat anything from "arthritis to digestive disorders such as diverticulitis to leaky bowel syndrome, viral infections, cold sores, bone pain, and it even cleanses the kidneys."[69] Since it's an anti-inflammatory and antiviral herb, it naturally helps boost your immune system to fight off infections. It also helps the body fight off free radical damage due to oxidative stress and cancers like breast and leukemia.

"A 2001 in vivo study demonstrated that the bark of cat's claw (Uncaria tomentosa) prevented the growth of the human breast cancer cell line MCF7 by having antimutagenic and antiproliferative effects on the cancer cells."[70]

Cat's claw can help maintain healthy cells and improve DNA by helping the body repair itself. On another note, it can improve and decrease high blood pressure because it contains hirsutine, which is an alkaloid. "This health-promoting alkaloid has been found to specifically act at the calcium channels of the heart and blood vessels as a calcium channel blocker."[71] This is important because, "Calcium channel blockers can lower blood pressure by blocking calcium from entering the cells of the heart and blood vessel walls. Calcium channel blockers also widen and relax the blood vessels themselves, which helps blood flow in a healthy, smooth manner."[71]

Suffer from Crohn's disease? Cat's claw can help reduce the inflammation caused in the gut and improve your overall digestive health. Lastly, it battles herpes and boosts your immune system by helping to increase the white blood cell count, which is known to fight off disease and infections.

Next time you're in your local grocery store, go over to the natural foods or vitamin section and grab a bottle of cat's claw!

CUCUMBER

Cumber is one of the bases in most detox waters, and it's great with hummus. From their crunchy exterior to their versatile and lightweight interior, cucumbers are excellent for weight loss, and they aid in dehydration, cognitive health, and much more.

Made of about ninety percent water and less than twenty calories per cup, cucumbers help you feel and stay full longer, which aids in overeating. They're full of vitamins and minerals that help detoxify the body by cleansing the liver, and since they're a natural diuretic, your urine will release any excess and unwanted toxins.

Ever wonder why you always see elder women putting cucumbers under their eyes? Due to the high vitamin C content, cucumbers, when applied directly to the skin, can reduce inflammation, swelling, and redness, and they can even treat acne. They are full of water, so that helps keep the skin and body nourished and refreshed to decrease chances of dehydration.

Cucumbers also help with blood pressure and overall heart function. They're full of potassium, which is known to lower blood pressure and manage fluid balance. Do you often eat a poor diet or struggle with maintaining proper bodily pH? Cucumbers help alkalize the blood by balancing the body's pH, which helps fight inflammation, infections, and several diseases common to individuals with high acidic diets. Cucumbers also contain magnesium, which can help relieve bloating, constipation, and even naturally clean or heal your gut.

Vitamin K deficient? Cucumbers contain vitamin K, which can help children and adults build and maintain strong bones. "Vitamin K builds strong bones better than calcium."[72] I know, shocking, right? Most adults are vitamin K deficient and don't even know it is due to lack of proper nutrition. However, if you start by eating cucumbers, you will be taking the first step to living a healthier lifestyle.

CRANBERRIES

Commonly known for preventing urinary tract infections (UTI) and a staple at Thanksgiving dinner, cranberries are not only sweet and versatile, they're packed full of nutrients and health benefits. Cranberries contain proanthocyanins, which help add hydration and prevent bacteria from sticking to the urinary tract walls, which, in turn, helps avoid infections. Cranberries are packed with vitamin C, vitamin K, and antioxidants. The antioxidants help fight against inflammation and fight free radical damage. Inflammation is usually at the root of all major health concerns.

Is cancer a big issue in your family like mine? Cranberries may help prevent certain cancers like prostate, breast, colon, and even lung because of their ability to fight off free radicals that may damage cells, as we mentioned earlier, and protect cellular structure and healthy cells.

Do you have severe allergies or manage to always catch every germ known to man? Cranberries contain polyphenols which help strengthen the immune system so you can fight off illness and infection. Also, the vitamin C and manganese they contain boost your immune system and combat nasty bacteria, promoting a healthy body system. Another interesting fact about cranberries is that since they help the urinary tract, they have the same effect on the digestive tract. Cranberries are an antibacterial and have detoxification properties. They aid in riding the body of toxins and unwanted pathogens. From upset stomach, buildup of acid, constipation, and GERD, cranberries help maintain healthy gut bacteria. Some even consider it a probiotic.

Lastly, cranberries can even help you maintain clean, pearly white teeth by riding your teeth of plaque and buildup. Of course, this is paired with brushing at least twice a day.

Try to eat cranberries whole. When cooked, this fruit starts to lose some of its health benefits.

CHICORY ROOT

Is it a tree or some form of bark? No, chicory root is actually an inulin, which is a pre-biotic fiber that aids in digestion, weight loss, inflammation, stress, and even diabetes. Chicory root helps the gut by promoting good bacteria, increasing the microbes in the gut for great bowel movement. It decreases constipation and softens stool. Plant polyphenols can combat inflammation, and since chicory root is a plant-based carbohydrate, it can help reduce chronic inflammation in the body. This is great for humans because most causes of diseases such as heart disease, cancer, and diabetes are due to inflammation.

Prediabetic or diabetic? A study done by the *Journal of Traditional and Complementary Medicine* showed that the level of adiponectin, a protein that regulates glucose levels as well as the fatty acid breakdown, significantly improved in those participants who had the chicory root extract. In essence, this means chicory root can have a beneficial effect on blood sugar and insulin resistance, which will help maintain balanced blood sugar levels.[73]

Lastly, chicory root has antioxidants, which help fight against free radical damage and protect the body's healthy cells and organs.

CASHEWS

You can make milk with them, make butter and—newly found—even cheese. They are packed with antioxidants, fiber, protein, and essential nutrients. From helping to prevent cancer, diabetes, and obesity, cashews are a versatile nut.

Cashews are great for improving cholesterol due to the compounds they contain that help with proper absorption of cholesterol. Furthermore, they help with oxidative stress and inflammation, which is known to help prevent heart disease and reduce the risk of plaque buildup in the arteries.

Suffer from depression or ADHD? Cashews are known to support proper cognitive function. They help keep the synapses firing and control neurotransmitter pathways.

Eating cashews can provide you with a boost of energy and speed up your metabolism throughout the day. Are you melanin deficient? African Americans are melanin rich; however, for lighter pigmented individuals, cashews can help with skin pigmentation due to their high copper content and even improve the skin's elasticity.

At risk for osteoporosis or osteopenia? Cashews are filled with vitamin K, potassium, magnesium, and calcium, which all can help maintain strong bones.

When it comes to weight loss, most individuals struggle with it, but cashews can help you overcome that battle. Yes, they are a fat, but they are a monounsaturated fat, i.e., a good fat, and they're nutrient dense. They help you feel full for a longer period, thus reducing constant snacking, and they curb those bad cravings.

Even individuals with diabetes can benefit from cashews. They have active ingredients that can stimulate glucose transport and control. Also, they "slow the rate at which blood is released into the bloodstream,"[74] therefore making them ideal for people who suffer from diabetes. Certain cancers such as colon, stomach, and digestive can sneak upon humans without warning. Cashews are great antioxidants that help fight these cancers. They contain phenols that help fight against cell and free radical damage.

Try them roasted, plain, as a cheese, or milk. Cashews are an excellent nut for the body!

CHLORELLA

Isn't that a fungus? Actually, it's an algae, and it's made up of about sixty percent protein and contains all the essential amino acids, making it a nutrient-dense food. Chlorella is full of iron and vitamin C. Not only does it help build your immune system to create antibodies to fight infections and unwanted pathogens, it also removes toxins from your body. From keeping your cholesterol levels balanced, to regulating blood sugar, improving lung function and respiratory health, to aiding in fighting off disease with high antioxidant content, chlorella is a superfood!

We all want to stay young or at least look younger, right? Chlorella is known to help you appear younger by decreasing stress on the body, which can age you rapidly.

Also, chlorella "naturally increases levels of vitamin A, vitamin C, and glutathione in your body, which eliminates free radicals and protects your cells."[75]

Last but surely not least, chlorella contains lycopene and chlorophyll, which may help "fight diseases such as HPV or human papilloma virus and even heart disease."[76]

So whether you choose to add it to your favorite beverage or take it straight, make sure this algae is part of your daily regimen.

CHAGA MUSHROOM

You may be thinking, *What in the world? I know about cremini and even shiitake, but what is a chaga?* Well, chaga mushrooms look like a rainbow. They're a type of fungus and are typically grown in cold climates. Full of antioxidants, these mushrooms fight against diseases. They can aid in slowing down the aging process because they help fight against oxidative stress, which is a precursor to the aging process. Also, since these antioxidants are present, they can help fight against cancer and help improve cholesterol levels.

We all know when we are stressed our blood pressure rises. Since chaga mushrooms help reduce stress, it, in turn, helps lower blood pressure. Furthermore, "Some research on mice suggests that chaga may help regulate the production of cytokines, supporting the immune system by helping cells communicate with one another. This could help fight infections, from minor colds to life-threatening illnesses."[77]

Chaga mushrooms may strengthen the production of T-cells and help the body fight unwanted bacteria and viruses.

Lastly, chaga mushrooms may increase your physical endurance by growing your glycogen or fuel levels. So next time you're in the supermarket, don't just run for cremini or shiitake mushrooms; grab some chaga!

BITTER SWEET HEALTH

Diabetes is big on my mother's side of the family, so growing up, we didn't get to have sweets or even chocolate. We received a homemade dessert once a week, but, little did we know, we were getting the good quality stuff because it didn't have preservatives. As you can guess, when I got older and was out of the house, I went crazy for chocolate! Yet milk chocolate was too sweet for me and it gave me severe acne breakouts, which are not a girl's best friend. One day, I was watching Dr. Oz, and he said, dark chocolate is actually good for you due to the antioxidants it contains. I did some research, and the next week, I went to the store and bought some. At first, the taste was too bitter, but a friend of mine told me I should combine the dark chocolate with milk chocolate to balance the taste until my palate adjusted. I gave it a try, and now, I only eat dark chocolate, and, guess what, no breakouts over here! The first thing I did was tell my mom and dad, and they made the switch as well. I am not pre-diabetic, my mother is not diabetic, and we stopped the cycle in our family by making a small change.

D

DATES

Although naturally sweet, with pits inside that can be removed, you can indulge in dates and not feel guilty afterwards. Dates can help reduce cholesterol, give you energy to last throughout the day, and help build strong bones. Rich in calcium and phosphorus, dates can give you strong bones and healthy tissues. The combination of both can repair body cells and maintain healthy bones and teeth.

Medjool dates are high in fiber and, therefore, help circulate the blood effectively through the body, helping to maintain great heart health. With high fiber content, these dates also help relieve constipation.

Have severe stomach pain and not sure of the cause? Eat some dates to see if you were just stopped up or if it's something more serious. Need a quick pick me up or just tired? Dates are full of nutrients to give you energy. Yes, they're high in sugar, but it is natural sugar; therefore, your body knows how to process it, unlike processed sugar.

Instead of constantly drinking coffee or an energy drink, try a few dates instead for that afternoon energy boost.

DRAGON FRUIT

It's not your typical or common fruit, but it's filled with benefits. Dragon fruit is not a fruit that dragons eat; instead, it's a tropical superfood. Packed with vitamin C and several B vitamins, dragon fruit can help you fight off the common cold and boost your immune system. Did you know dragon fruit has micronutrients that may help fight cancer? Due to the antioxidants present in dragon fruit, you can not only be healthy internally but externally as well. Phosphorus in this fruit promotes firm and tight skin along with vitamin C that provides a glow and younger look.[78]

Dragon fruit is high in omega fats, which can help your heart. Hundreds of thousands of people die every year due to heart disease or cardiovascular complications. It can help lower your triglycerides and overall cholesterol for a healthy heart and proper blood circulation.[79]

Also, dragon fruit contains properties that work as prebiotics to help with digestion and absorption to maintain a healthy gut. Furthermore, the high fiber content can relieve constipation and even decrease your risk of developing digestive issues such as diverticulosis.

Lastly, dragon fruit may help prevent certain cancers due to its lycopene content. According to a study done and published in *Nutrition and Cancer*, "Cancerous cells had difficulty living and were significantly reduced when treated with lycopene. Ovarian cancer evaluation showed a decrease in cancerous cell numbers after lycopene treatment."[80]

It may not be a common fruit you purchase at the store, but dragon fruit is definitely worth diving to find.

DILL

Most people only know dill when referring to a pickle, but dill is actually an herb. It can help alleviate menstrual pain and cramps, help with depression, increase your good cholesterol and even repel bugs! Dill is high in iron, antioxidants, and calcium, and it's an anti-inflammatory. Dill has been shown to aid in lowering cholesterol by decreasing the lipids in the blood and having a positive effect on the liver. Research has shown that dill, when in oil form and applied topically to the skin, can repel insects. The oil helps protect against insect bites and stored grain from insects.

Have you ever witnessed a person have an epileptic episode? It can be scary. Dill may help with seizures. "According to research published in the *Malaysian Journal of Medical Sciences*, the aqueous extract of dill leaves was reviewed for its effects on treating convulsions and epilepsy. The evaluation defined the plant as having a traditional medical reputation for profound anticonvulsant activities, potentially working as a natural alternative treatment for epilepsy."[81]

Dill has antioxidant properties and, thus, helps fight against inflammation and free radical damage. Dill weed has been shown to fight against bacteria and several fungi common to humankind. From mold to yeast and even candida, which is common in women, dill can help. So the next time you are thinking about grabbing a dill pickle, try grabbing some dill seed as well.

DARK CHOCOLATE

Chocolate, oh chocolate! Almost everyone loves chocolate, but is all chocolate unhealthy? Actually, no. Dark chocolate is packed with nutrients and antioxidants that help keep you healthy. Granted, it must be consumed in moderation, and make sure it has seventy percent or more cacao, which is the bean from which chocolate is derived.

From balancing your blood sugar to giving you a quick boost of energy, to maintaining a healthy heart, dark chocolate has amazing health benefits. Let's dive into a few. Free radicals damage the body and cause toxins to be present; however, the antioxidant properties in dark chocolate help fight and neutralize these radicals. Furthermore, dark chocolate is rich in flavonoids, which are plant compounds and known to help fight off certain diseases and health concerns.

Dark chocolate may also improve your heart's overall functioning ability and lower blood pressure.

Ever walk into a room and forget what you went in for, or maybe you have frequent brain fogs. Dark chocolate may improve your brain's ability to process information and retain it as well. According to a study from the *Journal of Nutrition,* "Intake of flavonoid-rich food, including chocolate, wine, and tea, is associated with better performance across several cognitive abilities and the associations are dose dependent."[82] Therefore, dark chocolate intake may help with brain function and cognitive ability.

Everyone dreads hearing what their cholesterol levels are. But did you know dark chocolate can help improve your overall HDL or "good" cholesterol and decrease your LDL or "bad" cholesterol? There are several different acids or healthy fats found in dark chocolate that can balance or neutralize your cholesterol, meaning it can increase your good and decrease your bad.

Dark chocolate may also fight inflammation and control your

lipids, so eating a small piece of dark chocolate can do wonders for the body.

Are you diabetic? Research has shown that diabetics who consume less than one ounce of dark chocolate per day with a high cacao count saw lower blood sugar levels over a period of time. Whether you want something sweet, you're watching your sugar levels, or you need an afternoon energy boost, grab a square of dark chocolate!

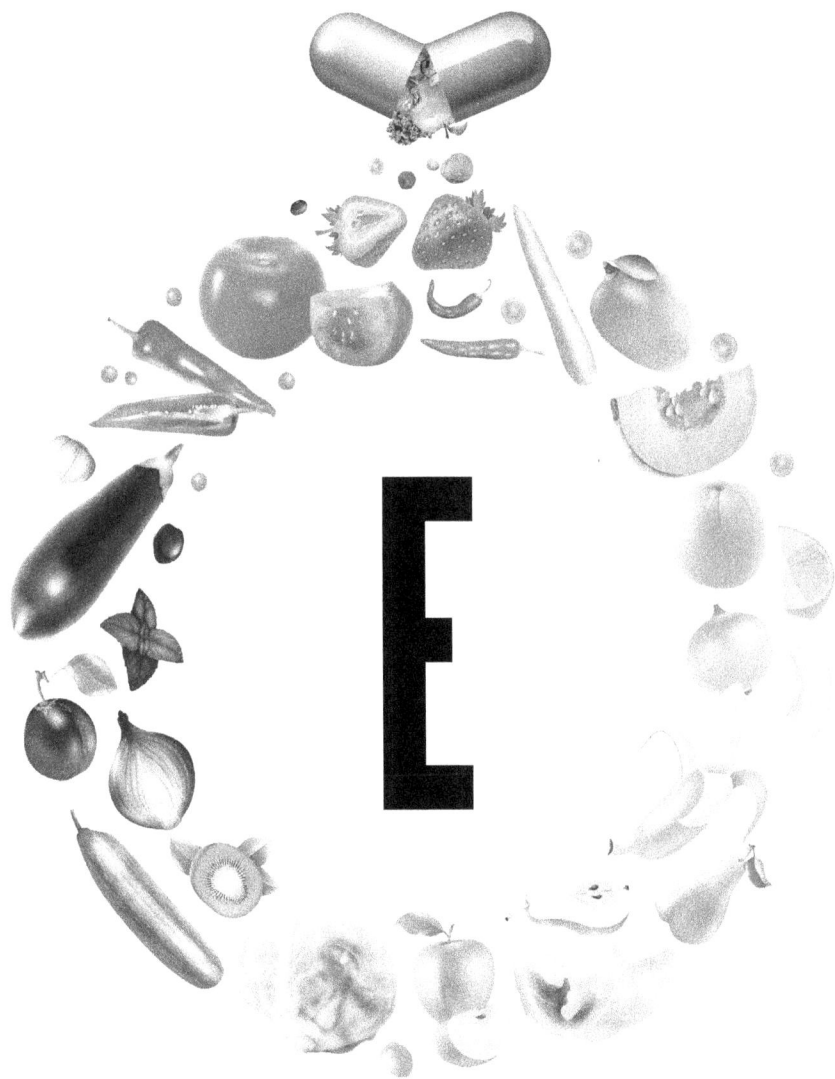

EGGPLANTS

A vegetarian favorite, eggplant has a deep, rich purple color and is versatile when cooking. Eggplant is known to have antioxidants and low carbs. It's low in calories and has anthocyanins, which give it its pigment. However, eggplant does much more for the body. Did you know cooking eggplant provides more benefits than eating it raw? The heat releases more health benefits from the plant. *Wow!* I know, just amazing! Eggplant contains an antioxidant in the skin called nasunin. Nasunin has been shown to fight free radical damage. Furthermore, it contains chlorogenic acid, which is "known to be very beneficial in stopping free radicals from forming cancerous cells and leading to cancer tumor growth."[83]

Eggplant has antimicrobial and antiviral compounds and helps reduce inflammation. It may even prevent disease and cancer cells from replicating. Eggplant is great at maintaining good cholesterol. As previously mentioned, it helps reduce inflammation, which is great for the arteries and can reduce oxidative stress. Eggplant is packed with phytonutrients that can reduce plaque buildup and improve overall blood circulation in the heart.

Looking to improve your gut health or need a good cleaning out? Eggplant is full of water and fiber, meaning it will help pull toxins and unwanted waste from your system all while making you feel fuller longer. The nutrients in the plant will keep your colon and digestive tract clean and prevent useless buildup, keeping inflammation down and helping to reduce your chances of developing diseases. Eggplant can also help you lose weight because it's packed with vitamins and nutrients, and it's low in calories.

Manganese is a mineral found naturally in the body but in a low percentage; therefore, we must obtain a good amount from food. Why am I telling you this? Eggplant is packed with manganese, which is needed to maintain healthy bone formation, connective tissue, and hormone regulation. It also helps use calcium effectively and makes enzymes that are needed for strong bones. It may even help stabilize healthy thyroid function, fight depression, and even control sugar levels.[84]

Feeling sluggish or down and need some energy to make it through the day? Eggplant can help! It is packed with B vitamins, from B6, which helps with blood regulation, making proteins, and giving energy, to B1, which helps keep your metabolism and brain healthy. Eggplant has you covered.

ELM BARK

Yes, you read that correctly—bark like on a tree. Granted, this is not just any bark. Elm bark can provide relief in many ways. From irritable bowel syndrome (IBS), to breast cancer, GERD, and even a sore throat, this tree bark is an often forgotten powerhouse. Slippery elm contains mucilage, a substance that becomes a slick gel when mixed with water, making a coating for the internal walls of the body to heal and reduce inflammation.

It contains antioxidants and may help regulate stool production and regularity. Furthermore, it possibly improves digestion and allows removal of unwanted waste and toxins at a faster rate, aiding in weight loss.

Deal with stress and feeling anxious all the time? Elm bark contains phenolics, which are compounds that guard against stress.

Fighting breast cancer? Slippery elm bark has been a go-to for several years to help alleviate pain and swelling from breast cancer. "When combined with certain herbs such as burdock root, Indian rhubarb, and sheep sorrel, it may improve conditions for women with breast cancer and improve depression, anxiety, and fatigue."[85]

The inner bark of the elm can be used topically to help treat skin infections, psoriasis, and eczema.

Elm bark is no regular tree bark; it is much, much more.

EGG

Eggs get a bad rep. One year, they were good for us, and the next year, we were told to avoid them. What is the truth about eggs? Well, both are true. It depends on the type of egg you purchase. Free range eggs are full of omega-3 fatty acids, which aid in preventing heart disease. Omega-3s help reduce inflammation, regulate and even lower cholesterol and, in turn, reduce your chance of developing heart disease.

Did you know eggs contain carotenoids? "Carotenoids act as antioxidants in the body and protect against harmful diseases, cellular damage, and aging."[86]

The most common food that contains carotenoids is carrots. However, eggs help absorb the naturally occurring carotenoids in vegetables and are great when paired with a diet high in green vegetables. Eggs are also beneficial for weight loss and eyesight. They help reduce your chances of developing glaucoma and macular degeneration because the carotenoid lutein, which is known to protect against retina damage, helps fight inflammation and works as an antioxidant. When it comes to weight loss, eggs are good due to their high protein content, which makes you feel fuller longer. Also, the lutein present in eggs may increase your physical activity level.

One interesting thing I've learned about eggs is that they contain choline. Choline is a macronutrient. We have to get it mostly from food because our bodies only produce a small portion of it. Choline is necessary for proper liver function, cognitive function, and brain development. One of the key things to check if you have poor liver function is if you are deficient in choline.

Lastly, eggs may help fight against skin cancer as well. Many people choose to eat avocados over eggs because they feel eggs are too high in fat; but you can still have your eggs; just omit the yolk and eat the whites.

EDAMAME

Typically, edamame is found at sushi restaurants and in Asian cuisine. Did you know edamame is just immature soybeans? So that's why they're green instead of tan or brown. Edamame is great for my vegetarians and vegans because they are high in protein and provide all the essential amino acids our bodies need. Edamame can even help with maintaining balanced cholesterol. *How?* They are packed with antioxidants and vitamin K, which help with your lipid profile, i.e. fats in the blood, which affects your cholesterol levels and helps reduce your chances of getting heart disease.

Edamame is packed with vitamins and minerals including folate, which we know helps with development, especially for babies in the womb. It's also packed with fiber.

Suffer from diabetes or are you prediabetic? Edamame can help lower your blood sugar because it contains low sugar, and it's low on the glycemic index. It's also low in carbs, which won't spike your sugar levels. So if you're watching your carbohydrate intake, this is an excellent snack choice.

As a soybean, edamame contains isoflavones, "a class of phytochemicals, which are compounds found only in plants. They are also a plant hormone that resembles human estrogen in chemical structure yet are weaker."[87] Therefore, they may help menopausal women with their symptoms and may even help reduce the risk of developing osteoporosis.

Eat them with salt cooked in the microwave. Boil them and pop them into your mouth, or go to your favorite restaurant and have them alongside your meal, but don't shy away from these baby soybeans.

ECHINACEA

Known mostly for its ability to prevent the common cold, Echinacea is good for so much more. It is a coneflower from Native America that can be used for medicinal purposes. From battling cancer, to internal pain, working as a laxative to even mental health, echinacea can do it all. When it comes to the common cold, Echinacea boosts and builds your immune system to fight the infection. Furthermore, taking echinacea at the first sign of a cold can reduce the longevity. It also helps relieve pain associated with headaches or sore throats.

Deal with a lot of stomach pain due to constipation and/or diarrhea? Echinacea can help bring you relief. It is known to provide a calming relief to the stomach, and it's a natural laxative. It may heal the intestines and stomach while also being an ant-inflammatory for the body. Echinacea, as an herb, can be made into a tea, and when drank regularly, it will calm the body down and relieve stress and anxiety, which will help with mental health and overall cognitive function.

Echinacea helps regenerate skin and produce healthy skin cells. So if you deal with eczema like myself or even psoriasis, echinacea should be your best friend.

From genital herpes, yeast infections, strep throat, and the flu, echinacea's anti-inflammatory and immune stimulating and boosting properties will have you feeling your best in no time! Make this herb part of your daily routine ASAP.

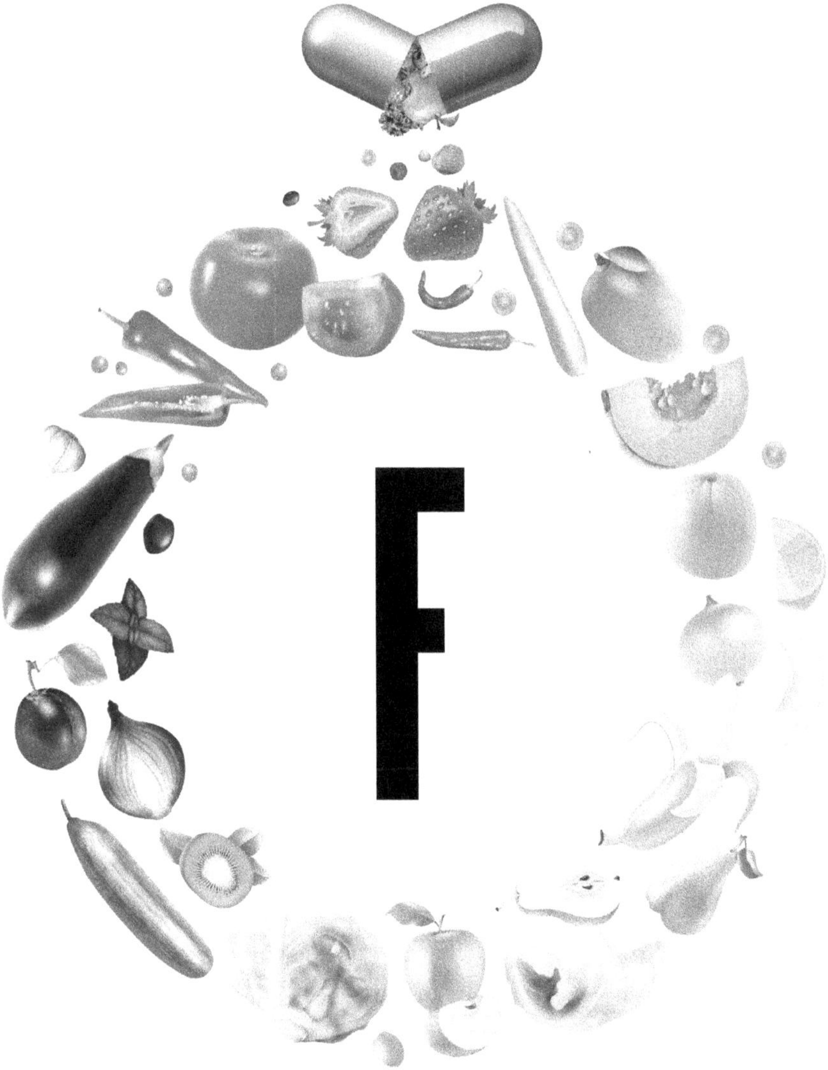
F

FENNEL

It's more than just a spice you use to season your food. Fennel is great for the immune system, high in fiber to improve digestion and can help the production of breast milk. Suffer from weak or frail bones? Fennel is great for bone health due to its high calcium. Not only can the calcium help, but the potassium found in fennel is crucial for your health as well. It's a great antioxidant because of the high level of vitamin C it contains, which helps fight free radical damage and promote healthy aging and skin.

Struggle with acid reflux or GERD? Fennel may help balance your pH levels in the body and digestive track to reduce reflux. It's low in sodium and, as stated previously, high in potassium, which aids in maintaining low blood pressure levels. Even when it comes to swelling or inflammation, fennel helps relieve excess water in the body.

For some parents, having a newborn can be exhausting if the baby has colic. Fennel seed oil can help improve movement in the small intestine and decrease pain for the baby, providing natural colic relief.

Cholesterol is a huge issue for thousands of Americans and fennel has been shown to help balance cholesterol levels. With the potassium and fiber it contains, it can lower levels, and it's great for overall heart health. "If you are on medication for your blood pressure, which may contain beta-blockers, you should avoid fennel since it is so high in potassium."[88]

So when you're doing your next weekly grocery store run, stop by the celery, grab that vegetable with the big white bulb, and make a great stir-fry.

FIG

Ever had figs? Growing up, my dad insisted his jam be made of figs. As a child, his mother made fig jam all the time, and he grew to love it. Little did I know, his love for figs would pass down to me. However, I never knew all the benefits they provided until I did a little digging.

Figs are packed with antioxidants that fight oxidative stress, and they're full of essential vitamins and nutrients for the body. Figs can boost your immune system; they contain antibacterial and antifungal properties that help fight off common sicknesses in the body. They are packed with fiber, which aids in digestion, lowers blood pressure, and makes you feel fuller longer. Eaten raw or dried, they are potassium and calcium rich, aiding in strong bones and body cells.

Figs can actually be healthier for you when dried properly versus eaten raw. Amazing, right? So run down to your local grocery store and pick up some figs today.

FENUGREEK

Fenu—what? Fenugreek is an herb, and it is highly known for its anti-inflammatory properties. It has numerous health benefits, but we will just cover a few. Since we know several diseases come from too much inflammation, fenugreek is essential in the diet. It has been known to help with digestive issues, from constipation to ulcerative colitis.

Women who have had a baby or did a little research about nourishing the baby may know how beneficial fenugreek is. It can help increase milk supply when breastfeeding. If you're struggling to produce adequate milk or your baby is hungry all the time (like my nephew) fenugreek acts as a galactagogue, which will stimulate milk supply tremendously.

Have a bad cough, chest pain, or bronchitis? Fenugreek can help relieve not only the pain but also the inflammation surrounding the ailment to get you back to optimal health in no time.

Did you know when something appears on the skin, it's your body's way of telling you something is wrong or off balance internally? For example: If you suffer from eczema, excessive rosacea, blisters, or even lots of dandruff, your body is informing you to pay attention and take action. You're in luck! Fenugreek can help decrease external inflammation as well, causing a decrease in all the aforementioned ailments.

Struggling to get it or keep it up? It's nothing to be ashamed of. Fenugreek can help. Although it is always best to consult your primary care physician before attempting to self-treat, fenugreek may increase sexual arousal and testosterone levels. Fenugreek has also been shown to increase sexual desire and performance in men.

FLAXSEED

Flaxseed is considered a superfood, and you can sprinkle it on oatmeal, add it to a smoothie, or coat your chicken with it. You may know that flaxseed promotes regular bowel movements and gives you added fiber, but it's way more beneficial than that. First, flaxseed is high in omega-3 fatty acids, and it's water soluble once digested. It contains ALA, or alpha-linolenic acid, which is known, according to webmd.com, to help prevent heart disease, lower blood pressure, and may help decrease cholesterol and even attempt to reverse atherosclerosis or the hardening of the blood vessels.

Some people are gluten sensitive or have celiac disease, and adding flaxseed to the diet is a great substitution for gluten. It is a good binder when baking and it's an anti-inflammatory, which is easy on the digestive system.

Just about every woman wants shiny hair, strong, long nails, and, of course, a smaller waist. Well, flaxseed can help with all those things. The B vitamins and fatty acids flaxseed provides can help your hair grow and remain itch and flake free. You can also apply flaxseed oil topically to your skin for a nice radiant glow, and these seeds can strengthen the nail cuticles.

I know, I know ... I didn't forget about the waistline. Since flaxseed is full of fiber, it helps you stay full longer throughout the day, thus making you take in fewer calories. Taking flaxseed will reduce inflammation due to its anti-inflammatory properties and excellent hormonal balance, which lead to weight loss and that ideal smaller waist.

Struggle with irregular periods or missed periods altogether? Flaxseed can help regulate your cycle by balancing your estrogen and overall hormone levels. Lastly, flaxseed is a superfood, meaning it's high in antioxidants, which have antibacterial and antiviral properties, so you may have fewer colds and get sick less throughout the year with regular consumption of flaxseed. It also helps rid the body of unwanted toxins and bacteria to maintain homeostasis in the gut.

While everyone else is on the chia seed kick, let's not forget about the original superfood seed—flaxseed.

FIT AND CONFIDENT

As a trainer, I interact and try to help a variety of people. One of my clients lost weight easily. He followed his meal plan exactly and trained four times a week; however, his entire body was fit, except his stomach. We cannot determine where we lose weight, but we can try our best to lose it in the places we want. He struggled with accepting his body this way and constantly complained to me about how unhappy he was with his stomach. I thought, *He doesn't have grapefruit in his diet; let's add it!* We added one cup of grapefruit to his daily regimen, and within three months, he lost five inches from his waist and an additional ten pounds overall. He was not only elated but had a newfound confidence I had never seen before. He thanked me profusely, and to this day, he has kept the weight off and loves his new body, including his mid-section.

G

GRAPEFRUIT

Grapefruit can range from very red, sweet, and juicy to tart and sour. The health benefits often get overlooked by other more common citrus fruits, but grapefruit is packed with nutrients and vitamins. Did you know grapefruit helps burn belly fat? I know, crazy, right! Of course, we already know that since it's a citrus fruit, it's packed with vitamin C and lycopene, but let's dive a little deeper and see how else grapefruit can help us out.

Struggling with weight loss or just want to speed up your metabolism? Grapefruit helps activate an enzyme in the body and may increase your metabolism to help you burn energy and fat.

Suffer from bad acne or hyperpigmentation? Your cure is here! Grapefruit helps with the production of collagen, which is essential for healthy and firm skin. Furthermore, the salicylic acid and lycopene it contains help prevent unwanted breakouts and skin damage. Also, it has been known to be an anti-inflammatory and help skin appear clearer due to bromelain, which is a protein-digesting enzyme typically used to remove dead skin and reduce inflammation in the body.

Instead of grabbing an orange when you're sick or have a cold, reach for a grapefruit. It's packed with vitamin C to help build your immune system and prevent future colds. Grapefruit may decrease the chance of developing certain cancers in the body due to the phytochemicals it contains. The antioxidant properties in grapefruit can help fight against free radical damage that is detrimental to the body and our DNA.

Lastly, grapefruit is low in calories, and if you pick a sweet one, you can help fight off those sugar cravings. Let's get a fruit bowl packed with oranges, lemons, and, now, grapefruit in all our homes.

GRAPES

Red, green, or black, seedless, seeded—What is your preference? The variety of colors of grapes serve different health benefits, and they taste different as well. I love the hard ones that pop in your mouth when you bite them.

We all know it's important to have a healthy heart and keep our cholesterol low, and grapes can help. "Consumption of grape products may have beneficial effects on the cardiovascular system by enhancing endothelial function, decreasing LDL oxidation, improving vascular function, altering blood lipids and modulating the inflammatory process."[89]

Everyone wants to live longer, right? I know I want to live forever! Grapes contain resveratrol, which is a plant compound that acts as an antioxidant, and it's found in the grape's skin. Resveratrol has been known to increase the genes related to lifespan.[90]

"California grapes were tested for their effects on glucose tolerance and inflammation and showed improved glucose tolerance and reduced inflammation. In addition, grape seed extract may prevent metabolic syndrome, type 2 diabetes, and obesity while improving gut health."[91]

Oxidative stress is one of the leading causes to several diseases we face as Americans. However, grapes are packed with antioxidants that fight against oxidative stress, and they help reduce severe inflammation in the body. Cancer is one of the major health concerns for a lot of people and families. Grapes may help prevent certain cancers. The skin of the grape is packed with nutrients and full of fiber, which may help with colon cancer. Furthermore, grapes, as an anti-inflammatory and antioxidant-rich fruit, can assist with breast cancer and pancreatic cancer.[92]

Wine gets a bad reputation, and many believe it's not good for you. To the contrary, wine is made from grapes, and red wine is beneficial for the gut and the blood stream. Did you know wine gets its different smells from the skin of the type of grape used to make it? Amazing! But, just as with anything, moderation is key.

The phytonutrients in grapes fight off unwanted bacteria and fungus within the body, ultimately leading to a healthy gut flora.

Now you can have grapes as part of your cheese board, as a midday snack, or even freeze them as a great healthy dessert option. Just make sure you eat them.

GUAVA

Grown in the wild in mostly tropical environments, guava is a powerful fruit for humans, and it can be eaten raw. This tropical fruit is inexpensive and packed with vitamin C. It contains *way* more vitamin C than an orange, and since our bodies can't store vitamin C, it is imperative that we get it through food. It is crucial for fighting off unwanted bacteria and preventing illness while promoting a healthy immune system.

Guava contains lycopene, which we commonly know is found in tomatoes, and we should eat those like candy; however, eating guava may help prevent cancer because it hampers the growth of the cells.

Guava is good for your digestive system as well due to the high fiber content. Fiber helps keep you feeling fuller longer, resulting in weight loss. Also, fiber helps remove unwanted foods and pathogens in the body, therefore helping to prevent constipation. According to draxe.com, "Guava fruit contains more antioxidants than almost any other fruit."[93]

Most Americans, especially African Americans, suffer from high blood pressure due to a high-sodium diet. Guava is packed with potassium, which helps fight against high sodium, decreasing your chances of developing high blood pressure. Calcium and potassium are essential for healthy bones, and guava's dense amount of potassium helps prevent bone loss.

Make a jam, eat it raw, purée it in a smoothie, or chew it as a dried fruit. Whichever way you like to consume your guava, just do it!

GINSENG

This root vegetable is found in a lot of Asian foods. It can help with fatigue and stimulate a positive mood in the body. Generally mixed with honey to make a tea or even diced to add favor to a dish, ginseng is great for not only taste, but can help us internally. So let's jump right in to find out how.

Ginseng is great for your overall health because it contains antioxidant properties and can help you lose weight naturally since it is an appetite suppressant. It may help prevent cancer due to its antioxidant properties and its ability to improve oxidative stress. It can also help hinder tumor growth and gene mutation.

Are you a smoker, or do you have poor lung airflow? Ginseng can help by reducing bacteria found in the lungs and improving overall lung function.

Diabetics, ginseng is for you! It may help reduce blood sugar levels when taken before meals and can assist with insulin sensitivity, according to a study done on Chinese medicine.[94]

A lot of men don't like to talk about this, but more men suffer from erectile dysfunction then we think. Ginseng helps stimulate the brain when it comes to sexual arousal and hormones and improves the central nervous system. Research done in 2002 at the Department of Physiology at Southern Illinois University's School of Medicine indicates that ginseng's ginsenoside components facilitate penile erections by directly inducing the vasodilatation and relaxation of the erectile tissue. It's the release of nitric oxide from endothelial cells and peri-vascular nerves that directly affect the erectile tissue.[95]

One of my favorite things about ginseng is its ability to prevent infections and illness and boost the immune system. From an early age, I've always had a weak immune system, so finding foods that helped boost my immunity was key. Ginseng has antimicrobial properties to help fight off unwanted pathogens, infections, and viruses. Furthermore, it can regulate our cells and decrease inflammation in the body, leading to a healthy overall body system.

There is a variety of types of ginseng, but the most common is white ginseng, and it can help improve your body immensely.

GINGER

The first thing someone may tell you to do when you're sick or have a cold is make tea, right? Once I became an adult, I started adding ginger to my tea. Why? Ginger is a huge anti-inflammatory and can help fight off disease, viruses, and infections. Ginger contains gingerol, which is "a pungent compound that may alleviate nausea, arthritis, and pain. Gingerols exhibit a host of biological activities ranging from anticancer, anti-oxidant, antimicrobial, anti-inflammatory, and anti-allergic, to various central nervous system activities. Inclusion of ginger or ginger extracts in nutraceutical formulations could provide valuable protection against diabetes, cardiac, and hepatic disorders."[96] Drinking ginger tea can boost your immunity and give you the extra push you need to start feeling better.

Ginger is affective at relieving nausea and upset stomach. *If ginger can help ease an uneasy stomach, maybe due to improper digestion, what about pain due to menstrual cycles?* Ginger is a winner in that department. Not only does it help reduce inflammation and bloating, ginger also eases the pain caused by menstrual cramps.

Whether you suffer from arthritis, sore muscles post workout, or temporary knee pain like myself, ginger should be a staple in your home.

Looking to shed a few pounds for the new year or just stay in shape? Ginger may help suppress your appetite and help obstruct fat absorption, resulting in a slimmer waistline.

As an additional benefit, ginger may balance your blood glucose levels and even help control your cholesterol numbers. Moreover, if you suffer from GERD or heart burn, ginger helps by reducing the overall stomach acid and inflammation causing the pain. Drink it in your tea with lemon, get it pickled at a sushi restaurant, or even candied at the grocery store. Whichever way you choose to take in ginger, just get it in.

GREEN TEA

Green tea has been known to help with overall energy and weight loss for years. But it also offers an enormous amount of substantial benefits. Let's take a look at just a few. Green tea is packed with antioxidants to help promote better health and improved vitality. It is great for your heart and blood flow because it aids in the pumping and flow of blood from the heart throughout the body, and it decreases the amount of work or pressure the heart undergoes. The antioxidants also help fight against free radical damage and can protect the brain against oxidative stress.

For people who are pre-diabetic or diabetic, green tea is essential for you. It can help balance blood sugar levels and even reduce your appetite, therefore increasing weight loss. Furthermore, green tea may help your body use more energy and increase your metabolism, resulting in a slimmer waistline. Ultimately, green tea can be taken in a pill form, or you can drink it hot or cold. Either way, it should be a staple for all.

Gingko

What is gingko? Its full name is gingko biloba. Native to China and Japan, Gingko is a tree, and there are several health benefits associated with it and even its leaves. First, it is packed with antioxidants that can help fight against free radical damage, known to cause several illnesses and diseases we see today. It is important for our hearts to work properly so blood flows adequately, but some suffer from poor blood circulation and have unhealthy hearts. Gingko can help due to its ability to increase blood flow by encouraging the dilation of the blood vessels. The increased blood flow may improve brain and eye health as well.

Is macular degeneration or glaucoma prominent in your family history? Gingko may help decrease your chances of developing these conditions. Good news, right?

Do you suffer from irritable bowel syndrome (IBS), chronic inflammation, or severe aches and pains around your joints? Gingko may provide some relief; it helps fight against inflammation and provides comfort and assistance.[97]

For COPD, bronchitis, bad coughs, and even asthma, gingko's anti-inflammatory properties may help improve air flow and overall lung capacity, allowing better breathing and lung health.

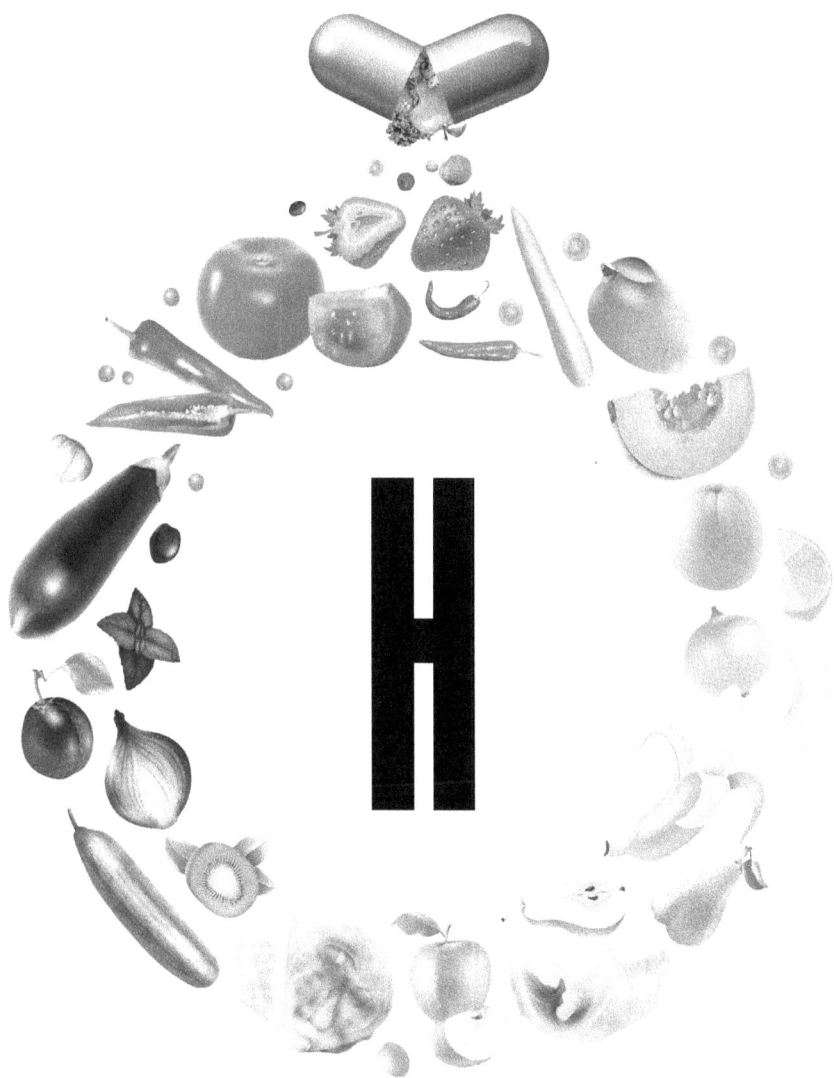

HONEY

It's made from bees. We use it in our teas and when baking or maybe to sweeten our favorite salmon dish. The type of honey you purchase can help your body fight against infections that affect your local area. Cool, right, but how? The bees in your local area pollinate from flower to flower, pulling the pollen and allergens in the area into their systems. The allergies we experience are local to our region. Therefore, when we purchase local honey made from these bees, it helps us build immunity to the allergens in our area.

Did you know there's different types of honey? With all the varieties of honey out there, what's the best one for you? Manuka honey is known to be the honey with the most health benefits. It's honey from bees that pollinate the manuka bush in New Zealand. Do you have severe stomach acid or suffer from GERD? Manuka honey is a natural antibiotic that fights against bacterial infections and can heal your body, especially your stomach. This honey may also fight against MSRA, a resistant strand of staph. "However, U.K. researchers from Cardiff Metropolitan University have offered us some natural hope. They discovered that Manuka honey downregulates the most potent genes of the MRSA bacteria. Some scientists now suggest that regular topical use on cuts and infections (especially in the hospital and nursing home setting) may keep MRSA naturally at bay."[98]

Manuka honey has antimicrobial, antioxidant, and anti-inflammatory properties, which promote healing internally and externally on the body. We all know that honey can help soothe a sore throat, but did you know manuka honey can help prevent the growth of bacteria that causes strep throat? It also helps with atopic dermatitis and acne when applied directly to the skin.

Suffer from sleep apnea or have always been a night owl? Manuka honey helps the body naturally release melatonin, which aids in a restful night sleep by allowing you to get into REM sleep or that ideal deep sleep.

Finally, this honey has been shown to help with digestion and inflammation in the intestines by repairing damage caused by free radicals and protecting against more damage in the intestines and colon. Granted, this honey is not inexpensive, but remember, you will pay for it now with your food, or you will pay for it later at the doctor's office. The choice is yours.

HIBISCUS

Known mainly as a flower and by several different names across the world, beautiful in smell and appearance, hibiscus is an undervalued plant. Did you know you can make it into a tea, and it has numerous health benefits? It may help lower blood pressure due to the high level of antioxidants it contains. Also, when taken consistently throughout the week, it may help balance and control blood sugar levels.

What about triglycerides and cholesterol levels? Hibiscus can decrease LDL levels and increase HDL to balance overall cholesterol.

Furthermore, it may fight free radical damage caused by oxidative stress because of the anthocyanins present, which give hibiscus its gorgeous color, and they even help to control metabolic syndrome.[99]

Are you a big red wine drinker? Maybe your favorite is cabernet or merlot. Hibiscus is compared to red wine because it helps encourage weight loss and weight management. It may even suppress or reduce the absorption of sugar intake when eating a meal.

I learned in my research that hibiscus may prevent NAFLD, which is non-alcoholic fatty liver disease. NAFLD occurs when there are too many fat cells in the liver not caused by alcohol use. "Hibiscus tea has been seen to benefit the liver by reducing the risk of this fatty buildup, which can potentially lead to cirrhosis, liver cancer, or liver failure if left untreated."[100]

Hibiscus is a natural diuretic that helps to relieve toxins and unwanted pathogens from the body. It may even help prevent kidney stone compounds in the bladder. Don't just think of hibiscus as a flower; consider its anti-everything properties and overall health benefits.[101]

HACKBERRY

These are not your traditional berries. You know about blueberries, raspberries, blackberries, and strawberries, but what about the hackberry? It's a pea-sized berry that comes from the hackberry tree, but unlike the other berries that are sweet in taste, the hackberry is tart, dry, and resembles a date. Though not a common berry, it does have some benefits.

Have a baby who is experiencing colic? The hackberry helps treat colic and aids in pain relief. Also, it helps with excessive bleeding during menstrual cycles and relieves diarrhea. Furthermore, the bark can be used to treat sore throats and venereal diseases.[102]

Lastly, it may regulate your period, and it's high in protein for my plant-based friends. Even though it's tiny, it's still beneficial, so don't overlook the hackberry.

HONEYDEW MELON

The green fruit. The other cantaloupe. You know, the melon. Often one of the most disliked pieces of fruit, honeydew melon is actually one of the best fruits for you. It is packed with B vitamins, potassium, and it can help you lose weight. Yep, now that you are paying attention, let's see what else this melon can do for us.

It's full of fiber and is made up of more than eighty percent water, so it will quench your thirst in the summer and keep you full, so eat away.

Suffer from constipation or excess calorie intake? Honeydew melon helps relieve constipation because its fiber pushes out unwanted waste, fat, and toxins from the body. And it's low in calories and gives your body the satisfied feeling nutritionally. Also, when it is picked at the peak of ripeness, it is super sweet, solving those sugar cravings in a healthy way.

Have you ever had a Charlie horse? That's because your sodium and potassium levels are off. Honeydew melon is packed with potassium, and it helps balance your body's electrolytes. On the other hand, it is vitamin C rich, which improves your immune system to help fight against sickness and disease. It also contains antioxidants that fight against free radical damage and promote healthy cell development.

Another advantage of vitamin C is that it promotes collagen production, aiding in healthy, glowing skin and fighting against cellular damage. Honeydew melon contains carotenoids just like carrots, which may assist in the fight against oxidative stress and unwanted pathogens. They also have anti-inflammatory properties and the carotenoids have chemo-protective properties, helping to protect healthy tissue.

Ever heard of atherosclerosis? *Athero-what?* It's a long word for clogged arteries. Honeydew can promote a healthy heart because its carotenoids combat free radical damage and protect our arteries.

This melon contains B vitamins, which are phenomenal for the brain and mood. They regulate our attitude and mood and can make us feel happy!

Honeydew melon also has folate, which is great for mom when she's carrying a child. It fights against folate deficiency and promotes adequate bone development and health.

Don't just think of it as the "sister" fruit to cantaloupe; honeydew melon is beneficial and can stand on its own. When you can smell its sweet aroma and hear a hollow sound when you thump it, you know you have a winner!

HEMPSEED

Hempseed can be made into an oil. It's an excellent plant-based protein and can even be applied directly to the skin and hair. "Hemp is a variety of the cannabis plant that actually has a long history of use in the United States. Unfortunately, since the 1950s, it has been lumped into the same category as marijuana because it contains a small amount of naturally occurring tetrahydrocannabinol (THC), and its use has been marginalized to a great extent. THC has been researched extensively, and science shows us that when it's not smoked, it has substantial health benefits."[103]

Hemp seeds are safe to eat and provide numerous health benefits for you and your family. Ladies, are you suffering from hormone imbalance or PMS symptoms? Hemp seeds contain gamma linoleic acid (GLA), which is a fatty acid substance that can help fight inflammation and hormone imbalance and promote cell growth when converted in the body.[104] This seed helps reduce pain from cramping and even migraines we may endure during our menstrual cycles.

Do you have a dry, flaky scalp, eczema like me, or even psoriasis? Hemp advances healthy cell growth and when converted to an oil, it penetrates deep into our second layer of skin, making it great for improving skin conditions and encouraging healthy hair growth.

When it comes to unwanted weight or wanting to shed those few extra pounds before a big event, hemp seeds can help due to their high fiber content, making you feel fuller longer. Also, they are a natural appetite suppressant, so when taken in the morning, you are less likely to feel hungry throughout the day.

They even promote a healthy gut and adequate bowel movements because of the combination of soluble and insoluble fibers they contain.

Lastly, hemp may boost your immune system and even keep your heart healthy by balancing your LDL and HDL level and improving your triglycerides.

Even though, for some time now, hemp was frowned upon, remember knowledge is power, and now that you know the benefits of hemp, don't hesitate to improve your health! Choose the seeds, oil, or both; your body will thank you!

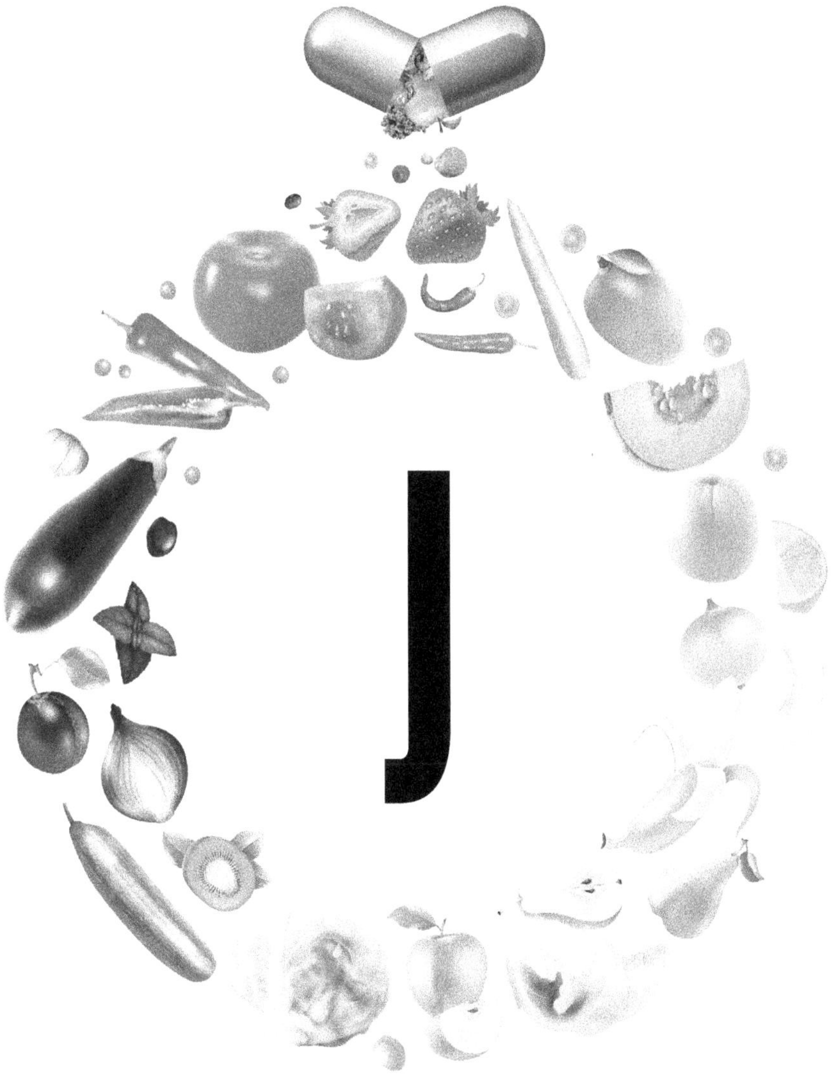
J

JACKFRUIT

Jackfruit is known for tasting like pork. It can be marinated and serve as a pork-substitute slider or eaten alone like pulled pork. It is vegan-friendly and really big in size. Find it in the fruit section at your local grocery store. *How is it beneficial and is it more than just a fruit that resembles pork?* Let's find out!

Did you know jackfruit is packed with calcium and magnesium? We know these minerals are necessary to have strong bones and healthy teeth, but our bodies lose calcium daily. So how do we replenish it? Our bodies absorb it from the foods we eat, which help us stay strong since we can't make calcium on our own. So if you suffer from weak bones, osteoporosis, or osteopenia, jackfruit is for you.

Black women are at risk for developing a form of magnesium deficiency, but eating about one cup of jackfruit weekly may help reduce the probability. Furthermore, jackfruit is packed with vitamin C and antioxidants to help your immune system stay strong.

It may help fight against free radical damage as well, and the antioxidants will help ward off unnecessary toxins and pathogens in the system.

Jackfruit contains vitamin B6, which helps decrease your chances of developing heart disease. Vitamin B6 also assists the body in making melatonin, which helps us get better sleep. This vitamin even helps with brain development and function. Lastly, the strange seeds we see in jackfruit are essential, too, because they are packed with fiber, which will help you feel fuller longer and relieve you of an upset stomach or constipation.

It's not just an ugly or huge piece of fruit. It's a nutrient-dense meat substitute that is great for all individuals, young and old alike.

JICAMA

Jicama is a root vegetable. Growing up, I was always told it tasted like a mix between an apple and a pear. Now, I like frying it or making it into a tortilla for a low-carb option. You can eat it raw or cook it, and since it's made of mostly water, it's great for dieting or lifestyle changes, even people who are trying to watch their sugar levels.

Jicama is a high-fiber vegetable and great for digestion. "Jicama's fiber contains a beneficial type of prebiotic fructan carbohydrate called oligofructose inulin. Because it's indigestible within the human digestive tract and ferments in the gut, inulin is considered to have zero calories, yet it benefits the digestive organs and, therefore, your entire body Z(including the immune system) in a few different ways. Inulin acts like a prebiotic once it reaches the intestines, which means it helps probiotics (or 'good bacteria' living within the GI tract) do their job best."[105] This helps the body control and increase weight loss and improve overall digestion.

Suffering from diarrhea, constipation, or IBS? Because jicama is packed with fiber and it's a water-dense vegetable, it helps relieve and treat the aforementioned ailments and reduces pain or reactions caused by inflammation in the gut. Jicama is also known for inhibiting the appearance or replication of unwanted cells or growths that can turn cancerous in the body and digestive system. The digestive system is big on having an adequate balance of good and bad bacteria, and jicama keeps the system in homeostasis to aid in proper functioning. Jicama contains vitamin C, which supports a healthy immune system and fights free radical damage and even oxidative stress. Its potassium aids in reducing inflammation in the body, and it's also great for the heart. It may reduce cholesterol levels, and we already know it helps balance blood sugar. Those two benefits combined can help decrease the appearance of metabolic syndrome.

Lastly, jicama is great for healthy bones. Its magnesium content fights against bone degradation and assists in the support of bone mineralization in the body. Ideally, this vegetable is perfect for older individuals who may suffer from bone loss, but everyone can benefit from jicama to prevent bone loss and increase bone density.

JAMBOLAN

Jambolan is a tree, and all forms of it can be used to help heal the body. If you suffer from diabetes or you're pre-diabetic, the jambolan seed is ideal because it may help lower blood sugar levels in humans. Have severe upset stomach, ulcerative colitis, or diarrhea? Jambolan can help ease the pain and possibly decrease your chances of developing those ailments.

Do you struggle to get into the mood? Surprisingly, many people do, and you are not to worry because jambolan is known as an aphrodisiac to aid in jumpstarting those sexual desires. Jambolan also helps fight against unwanted swelling and severe inflammation and may even protect against oxidative stress.[106]

Whether you struggle with bowel movements, blood sugar, or getting in the mood, jambolan can help. It can be found at your local grocery store.

JASMINE

Jasmine is a flower, and no, you can't eat the flower for the benefits; instead, you can get the oil from the flower. Jasmine oil can help aid in depression relief, anxiety, stress, and pain from childbirth. It also assists you in getting a good night's rest. Let's see how this is possible and what other benefits this oil contains.

Jasmine oil can increase your energy levels by the way it activates the brain. It contains a stimulating effect on the brain to give you that extra boost.

Suffer from sinus infections, allergies, or frequent runny noses? Jasmine oil has antimicrobial and antibacterial properties to fight against infections and illnesses. Place this essential oil around your home to keep a clear nasal passage and increase your immunity.

The dreaded menstrual cycle is something most women never look forward to. From PMS symptoms to overall exhaustion, it's no fun. Jasmine oil may balance our hormone levels and relieve some of our symptoms. Jasmine oil may help balance hormone levels by acting as phytoestrogens, plant constituents with a phenolic structure similar to estrogen. This gives therapeutic-grade oils, including jasmine oil, the ability to help correct PMS, menopause and other hormone-related issues.[107]

If you are like me, you're often tired but have trouble falling asleep at night. Well, here is our relief! Jasmine oil has a calming and relaxing effect on the body, much like medicine you can take to help you sleep, easing you into a good night's rest.

Now, most oils are great for your skin, and jasmine oil is no different. If you suffer from dry skin, eczema, wrinkles, or unwanted blemishes, jasmine oil helps revitalize the skin, balances oily skin, and brings a glow to the skin like never before.

So even though the flower is gorgeous, when you think of jasmine, also think of the wonderful benefits the oil can bring you.

JUNIPER BERRY

Just like all other berries, juniper berries are deep in color and rich in flavonoids and antioxidants, which fight against infections. Ideal for fighting illnesses, juniper berries help strengthen the immune system and improve respiratory conditions. We all have heard that cranberries are a great fruit to flush the body and aid with urinary tract infections (UTI), but juniper berries are great for that as well. They contain antibacterial components that make them ideal for flushing the body of toxins. Juniper berries can also be made into an oil and serve as an astringent and natural moisturizer for the skin and aid in relief of the itching and redness that's commonly associated with eczema and acne.

If you suffer from slow bowel movements, juniper berries may help because they stimulate digestion. "You can also use juniper oil as a cellulite remedy. It may help to reduce the appearance of cellulite thanks to active components like alpha-pinene, sabinene, and juniperene. Add 100 percent therapeutic-grade juniper berry essential oil to grapefruit cellulite cream to decrease cellulite."[108]

Not only do these berries help us internally, but they are great for external use as well. Did you know juniper berry oil is a natural antiseptic? It has antibacterial and anti-fungal properties, making it a great home cleaner and good for topical use.

It also gives off an aroma that insects can't stand, making it the ideal bug repellent. When made into an essential oil and placed on the body, it can help us de-stress and provide a calming sensation throughout.

Lastly, placing it in the home as an aroma to inhale can assist with sleep deprivation and reduce overall anxiety. Use it on the body, in the body, or in the home. Just don't overlook juniper berry and its significance.

JOJOBA

The first time I heard of jojoba was from my sister, who is a naturalista (a woman who keeps her hair in its natural state), and she told me it's great for your hair. So I did a little digging to learn about jojoba. Jojoba is a plant, and the oil from the plant is a wax. Wow! This oil is not just good for hair, but it also promotes healthy skin and can fight infections, just to name a few benefits. Let's examine a few other areas where this plant can help us.

Have oily skin, dry skin, or eczema? Jojoba oil acts as a lubricant to protect the skin and keep it moisturized. It also helps balance our glands to prevent producing too much oil, therefore preventing overproduction of oil in the skin and decreasing our chances of developing acne due to clogged pores. Jojoba oil is great for the skin also because it aids in the healing process when we get cuts or bruises. It decreases the presence of wrinkles and stimulates collagen production and synthesis.

If you are like me, you hate taking your makeup off at night because you have to wash your face like three times before it completely comes clean. Well, if you apply a small amount of jojoba oil to a cotton ball, your makeup will come off with ease.

Jojoba oil contains vitamin E, which has antioxidant properties and helps decrease unwanted inflammation in and on the body. It can help treat a burn from the sun or an accidental burn in the kitchen by speeding up cell healing and regeneration while soothing and moisturizing the skin.

I mentioned infections, but what kind of infections does jojoba treat? From a toenail infection to a cut, athlete's foot or even warts, jojoba oil can help rid the body of unwanted pathogens with its antibacterial and antifungal properties. Do you suffer from split ends, alopecia, or a dry, flaky scalp? Jojoba oil helps moisturize and stimulate the hair follicles in the scalp, which leads to healthy hair growth. It leaves a shine and softens the hair, causing less breakage. It eliminates frizz when used regularly, and when it's applied directly to the scalp, it acts better than a conditioner, detangling and moisturizing the hair.

Jojoba oil even fights against free radical damage and oxidative stress with the B vitamins it contains. I guess my sister was right; she knew a little something about jojoba oil, but now we know way more.

HURDLES AND HEALING

In 2017, I was doing hurdles, and I came down too hard and suddenly stopped, causing a grade-two tear of my LCL in my left knee. When I went to the doctor, he wanted to perform surgery, but I felt it wasn't completely torn. *I can fix this,* I thought. I informed the doctor of my decision to heal my knee myself and not have surgery, primarily because I felt I was too young to have knee surgery. I did a lot of research, and after three and a half months, I was able to walk again by means of eating foods like kiwi, kale, and lean fish, which are high in vitamin C, fiber, and protein and low in fat. These foods are known to help repair tendons and ligaments in the body. I did my own physical therapy daily, gradually stretching and doing low-resistance exercises to build strength in my knee. I now run sprints and do hurdles, box jumps and more, all without having surgery or even medication—just food!

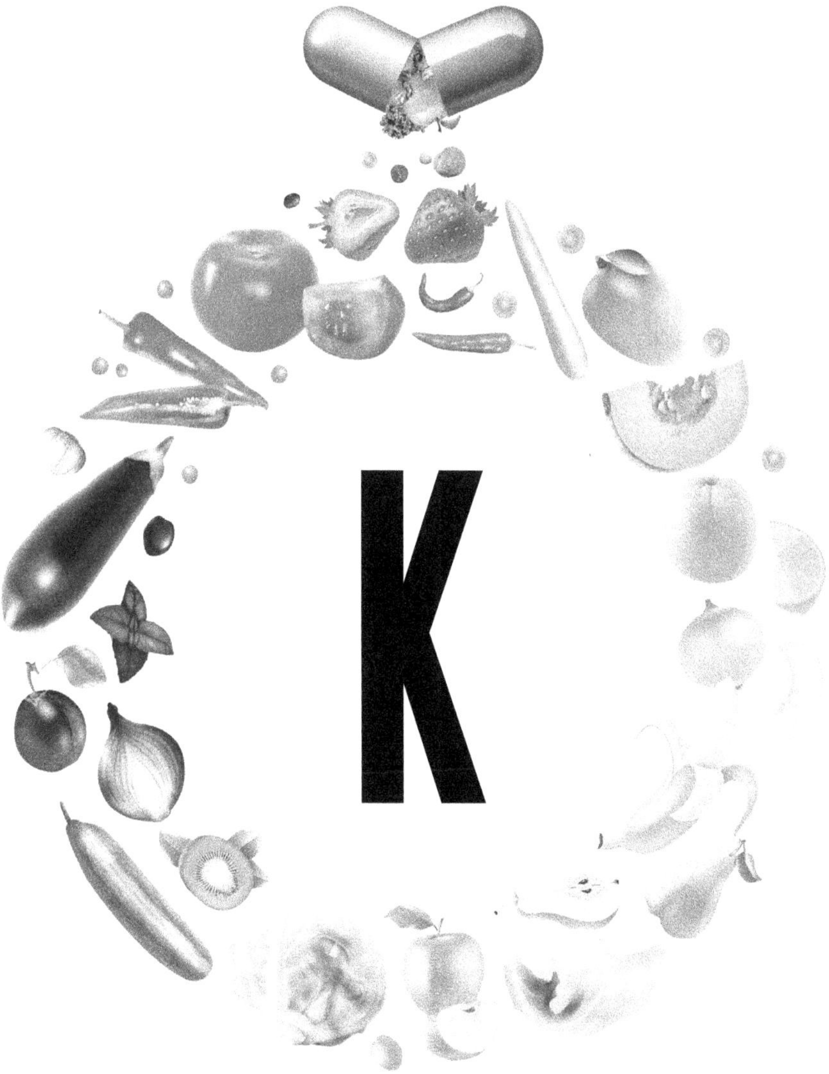
K

KEFIR

Have gut issues or lack enough probiotic intake? Kefir is a cultured dairy product that is packed with probiotics to aid in overall gut health. Kefir can be made from any milk, dairy or non-dairy, so it's safe for those who are dairy intolerant or sensitive. The kefir made from traditional milk is great for bone density and improving the strength of bones due to its high calcium level.

The older we get, the more at risk we are for osteopenia or osteoporosis and some even suffer from vitamin K deficiency, which leads to increased bone loss and bone degradation. Kefir contains vitamin K and may improve bone density, bone health, and absorption of nutrients in the body. Also, kefir is a "good probiotic" in that it fights against unwanted bacteria and protects against harmful toxins.

Is cancer prominent in your family? Do you know someone who has suffered from breast cancer? Kefir can play a great role in combating the disease. "It can slow the growth of early tumors and their enzymatic conversions from non-carcinogenic to carcinogenic, potentially stopping the spread of cancerous cells throughout the body."[109]

Furthermore, kefir builds the immune system and decreases allergic outbreaks due to everyday allergens because it helps change the way the body responds to toxins in the air, thereby suppressing the irritation.

When there is a problem inside the body, your system sends you signals to inform you something is not right. Do you have eczema or psoriasis? Kefir can help improve your skin by aiding the body's internal balance, causing skin irritations to decrease. Kefir also serves as a Band-Aid in that it increases wound healing and aids the integumentary system.

You ever get sick for more than a week, leaving you feeling weak and your stomach aching? What about irritable bowel syndrome (IBS) or Crohn's disease? When we're sick, on prescription drugs for an extended period of time, or have an unhealthy diet, we begin to break down and destroy the good bacteria in the stomach, which leads to poor gut health. Thankfully, there's kefir to the rescue! Kefir helps restore gut balance, providing good gut flora to fight against unnecessary germs and pathogens that may enter the digestive system.

Because there are live active cultures in kefir, it has to stay refrigerated, but you do not have to be a dairy drinker to enjoy kefir; there are options available for everyone.

KIWI

When we get a cold, the first thing we want is vitamin C to build our immune systems, so we may grab an orange; at least that's what I was taught as a child. But did you know kiwi contains *more* vitamin C than an orange? Kiwi is full of great nutrients and benefits, so we're going to examine just a few to get you to reconsider your next fruit of choice.

Kiwi contains vitamin K. *Great, what does that have to do with me?* Well, vitamin K is needed to regulate and metabolize calcium, and we all know calcium promotes strong and healthy bones. Everyone thinks milk provides those strong bones, but its more than the milk doing the work. If you're up in age or at risk for osteoporosis or osteopenia, kiwi is full of vitamin K and a great addition to your fridge.[110]

Kiwi is packed with antioxidants and low in calories, which is great for the digestive system and for those watching their waistlines. It also has antibacterial properties to fight off illness and unwanted microbes.

Kiwi helps reduce inflammation in the body and aids in proper bowel movement, reducing the risk of irritable bowel syndrome (IBS) and constipation due to its high fiber content.

Did the doctor inform you of elevated triglyceride levels, or are you just trying to keep an eye on your cholesterol? Kiwi is great for the heart because of its potassium and helps balance our potassium and sodium levels to maintain homeostasis in the body.

The vitamin C it contains helps heal, strengthen, and restore any internal and external damage to the body along with its tissues. It also helps us fight off free radical damage we experience daily, and it contains vitamin E.

Vitamin A is great for overall vision and eye health, and vitamin C helps the skin because of its collagen dependency, giving us a decreased chance of developing glaucoma or any blockage of the retina while giving us glowing skin and strong tendons and ligaments.

The next time you get the common cold, don't reach for the orange; grab a small, furry kiwi to get back to feeling like yourself.

KUMQUAT

Just think of it as a mini-orange, packed with vitamin C and nutrients. Kumquats are low in calories and high in fiber. The skin has a distinct flavor—Yes, you can eat the skin of this citrus fruit. It's relatively sweet, and the inside is tart. The fiber it contains helps keep you feeling fuller longer, aiding in weight loss and improved digestion.

Whether you suffer from irritable bowel syndrome (IBS) or frequent constipation, kumquats can provide relief by moving the stool through the system, reducing inflammation and irritation in the body. They are also rich in antioxidants, which fight against free radical damage and help prevent oxidative stress and damage to our cells. These antioxidants ward off infections and fight against bacteria and unwanted parasites we may encounter from the environment.

Kumquats are rich in vitamin C, which helps boost our immune system, reduce our risk of developing illness or the common cold, and may even improve our symptoms once infected. Eating foods with vitamin C and antioxidants can help reduce the risk or prevent the formation of certain cancers.

Known to South Asia, kumquats may be tiny, but they are mighty. Look for them in the organic produce section at your nearest grocery store. And remember, the skin is thin, so get it in!

KALE

Growing up, I couldn't wait until it got a little cold outside because my mom would make greens and cornbread. Yes, I am a southern woman, and I love greens and cornbread. The only greens I ever knew were mustards, collards, and turnips. My mom never cooked kale. When I became an adult, all I heard was "kale this" and "kale that." So I wondered what was this "kale," everyone was talking about. I came to find that kale is a green, too; it comes as a flat leaf or curly, and it's packed with health benefits!

Kale is full of antioxidants, which fight off free radical damage. There are several toxins and pollutants in our homes and outside, and we can't avoid them; however, antioxidants help fight against the damage they cause. Also, kale fights inflammation we suffer in the body, and as we learned earlier, chronic inflammation is the primary cause of several diseases and illnesses.

We know the deeper and richer the color of a vegetable the better it is for you, and the same applies for kale. It is packed with vitamins A and K and folate, which helps balance cholesterol and is excellent for maintaining overall heart health. Folate, as we know, is much needed for expecting mothers and infants because it aids in helping to prevent birth defects and improve brain development.

On the other hand, kale may also help prevent cancer. "Cruciferous vegetables contain glucosinolates, which, in broken-down form, are active compounds that have been studied and examined for their anticancer effects."[111]

Kale is great for riding the body of unwanted enzymes and toxins. This is a benefit because it may aid in weight loss by eliminating these toxins and preventing the formation of further toxins.

Granted, kale has a bitter taste when eaten raw, but you can cut the bitterness with a little acidity like lemon juice. You can put it in a smoothie, a salad, or even bake it into chips. Kale is a versatile green with many benefits to the body.

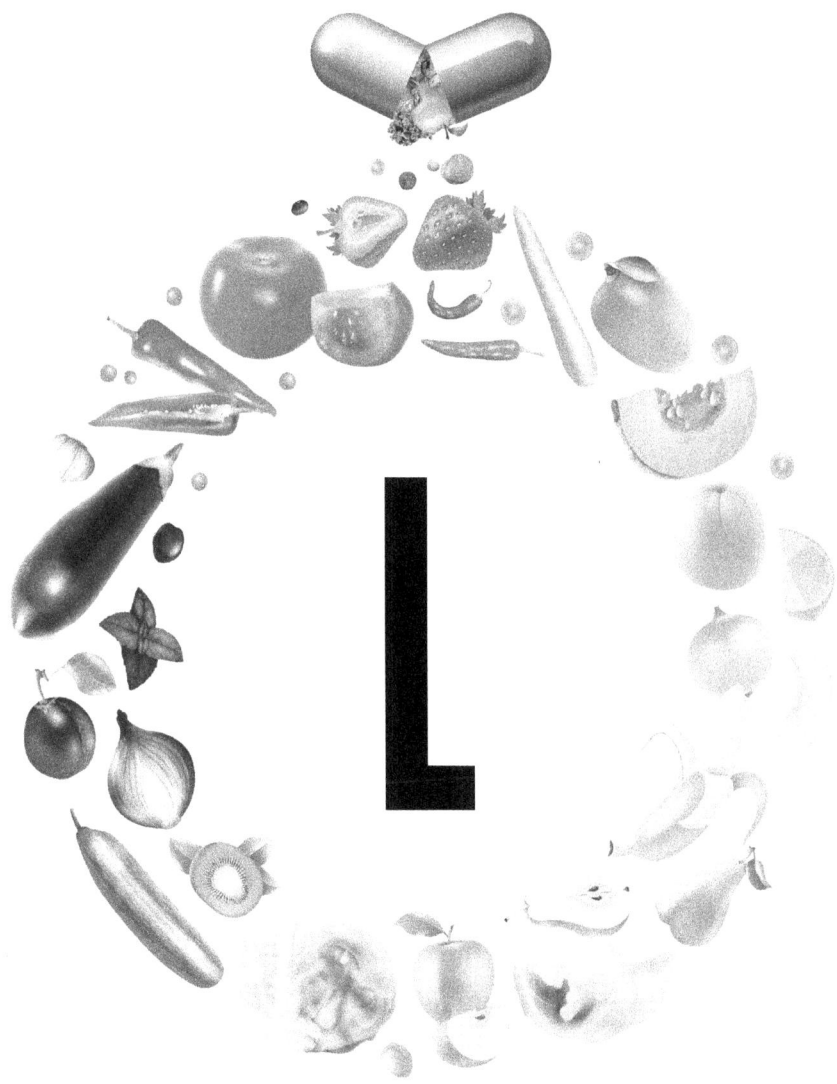

LYCHEE

Is this what we use in desserts? No, wait, I know, it's that thing vegans make to taste like pork! No, actually, lychee is a small fruit that belongs to the soapberry family and is native to China. You can get it fresh at the store or in a can, and you can use it while baking or for traditional cooking.

Lychee is packed with antioxidants, which help fight free radical damage and prevent and reduce oxidative stress on the body. Furthermore, lychee is packed with vitamin C, which we know helps ward off infections and diseases and helps build and maintain a strong immune system, reducing the reoccurrence of illnesses. Did you know we naturally have inflammation throughout our bodies? Granted, it's not a lot and it isn't substantially harmful; however, chronic inflammation is the root cause of most diseases today and can be extremely damaging. Lychee helps fight and decrease chronic inflammation and thwart free radical accumulation.

Not only is lychee an anti-inflammatory and antioxidant, but it also has antiviral properties that help decrease the spread of unwanted viruses throughout our bodies and to other people we encounter.

If you suffer from high blood sugar or your blood sugar has constant spikes and drops, lychee can help you. It is known for balancing blood sugar levels because of the fiber it contains. The fiber keeps you fuller longer, aiding in decreased food intake, and it slows the absorption of sugar into the bloodstream, keeping an overall balance.

Even though lychee is considered a tropical or exotic fruit, it can be found in the United States, and the best time to find it is in the summer months when it is in peak season.

LEMON

In recent years, many people have learned more about the health benefits of lemon. Traditionally, lemon was known for just being a garnish on fish or hanging on a glass of water. But as society has delved more into nutrition, we realize lemon is great for the skin, our organs, and even our hair. Let's get a little more specific and see how lemon can benefit us.

Fruits and vegetables rich in vitamin C have been known to improve heart disease and may even decrease your chances of developing high blood pressure. Since we know lemons are packed with vitamin C, they should be one of the top choices when focusing on overall heart health.

Wait, what if you're allergic to citrus like me? Don't worry, kiwi, as we learned earlier, is packed with vitamin C and can be an excellent substitute. Lemons may help fight certain cancers such as breast and prostate, and it inhibits cancer cells due to its cancer compounds like hesperidin[112] and d-limonene and its antioxidants.[113]

Whenever you get sick, the first thing you grab is tea, right? Usually in that tea is lemon and honey, but why? Lemons are full of antioxidants that help fight against free radicals and unnecessary pathogens and viruses. With loads of vitamin C, lemons help boost your immune system while decreasing inflammation throughout the body.

Do you suffer from kidney stones and ever wondered how to get rid of them? Lemons have citric acid, which is a compound, and that's what makes lemons tart. It also increases urination and filtering in the body and, in turn, can help prevent the accumulation of kidney stones.

I mentioned that lemons are beneficial for the skin, but how? When we get older, we start to age, which manifests wrinkles, sagging skin, and spots caused by free radical damage and buildup of unwanted pathogens. Lemons are full of antioxidants, which help fight radicals and oxidative stress and damage. Therefore, lemons are great for improving the skin and giving you that natural glow.

Are you iron deficient? Is it because you're not taking in enough iron, or is it because your body isn't properly absorbing the iron? Vitamin C is an excellent addition that will aid your body in adequately absorbing your iron intake. Lemons are a great choice to help prevent iron deficiency since they contain over seventy-eight percent of the daily value of vitamin C in one serving.

Lastly, lemon water is an ideal option for weight loss as a refreshing beverage choice instead of juice or soda. From kidney stones, to glowing skin, and even weight-loss, lemons are a wonderful addition to a healthy lifestyle.

LOQUAT

It's a small orange fruit with thin skin, native to the Chinese culture. Loquats are low in calories but high in nutrients. They're loaded with vitamins A, C, and B, calcium, iron, potassium, and many more vitamins and nutrients. Let's get specific about how it helps us. It's high in iron, which is helpful to all humans but especially women. Iron is needed for our red blood cells. Not only does it help prevent anemia, but it also boosts our circulation and energy.

The American diet is filled with sodium and saturated fats, which are harmful to the body as well as the heart. Loquats contain potassium, making it excellent for the cardiovascular system as it decreases pressure on the heart, arteries, and veins, resulting in lower blood pressure. Loquats also regulate blood sugar levels and help maintain sugar level balance, reducing the number of spikes and drops. Loquats can be made into a tea to help relieve phlegm in the throat and chest.

Loquats are viewed as expectorants, which promote the secretion of sputum by the air passages, used to treat coughs. Along the same lines, loquats are full of vitamin C, so they help build our immune system, aid in repairing our tissues, and even stimulate white blood cell production. Our bodies use white blood cells to protect us when we encounter foreign pathogens and germs.[114]

Not only does loquat work as an antioxidant, but it's also full of fiber, helping to maintain good digestive health and bowel movements as well as decreased weight loss and constipation.

Loquats can be enjoyed as part of a meal or as a snack. Just remember, don't eat the seed due to the toxic compounds it contains!

LONGAN

Similar to rambutan and lychee, longan is a tree that produces fine fruit. The longan fruit is small, almost translucent in color, and wrapped in a brownish shell or skin. The taste is close to a grape, and it's about the size of an olive. Even though it's small in size, it's large in benefits. Longan berries contain vitamin C, which helps fight against infections and strengthen our defense system for future encounters with bacteria. Vitamin C is also needed to properly absorb iron in the body. Longan is full of potassium, B vitamins and antioxidant properties. It can help reduce and may even prevent anemia since it contains more iron than meat and spinach.

It is great for improving the appearance of wrinkles and even those bags we get after long nights because of the nutrients it possesses. Lastly, it is excellent for the heart because it improves blood circulation throughout the body and may reduce your chances for heart attack or stroke.[115]

It's low in sugar, contains no fat, and it's low in calories, which is great for when you're watching your waistline and you want something sweet. Longan berries can be eaten fresh, dried, as a snack, or as an addition to a meal.

L -LYSINE

L-lysine is an amino acid that has been known to help treat the herpes simplex viruses. It can be found it foods because our bodies do not produce it, and it's useful in many ways. Do you suffer from cold sores often or always get fever blisters when ill? L-lysine, when taken at 1000 mg daily, has been shown to decrease the frequency and amount of cold sores on the body.

Always overwhelmed with anxiety or have constant stress from your job, home life, or other uncontrollable factors? L-lysine may be able to reduce your anxiety and stress levels and even manage cortisol levels in the body when taken daily.

Furthermore, L-lysine helps protect your bones by controlling and maintaining calcium in the body while increasing the overall absorption of calcium in the kidneys.

Many people do not know this, but L-lysine can help you heal faster from a cut or injury by aiding in collagen formation, therefore accelerating the healing and repair process in the body.[116] It can also act as a binding agent promoting the production of new cells and blood vessels.

You can purchase L-lysine in the pill form to give it direct access to your blood stream, or you may use it as a supplement through foods like salmon, tuna, and leeks.

LUTEIN

Lutein is an antioxidant found in deep-colored foods, especially those that are orange in pigment. It has been known as the "eye healing" antioxidant. It is an anti-inflammatory, which helps fight against oxidative stress in the body and unwanted pathogens.

Do you work outside, and the sun is always in your eyes? If so, lutein is great for you. It can fight against the damage caused by the sun that usually leads to cataracts or macular degeneration.[117] Do you like being in the sun or getting that wonderful tan, but you're concerned about skin cancer? Lutein may help prevent skin cancer by helping to sort the sun's strong wavelengths, thus decreasing the possible damage to the skin and overall stress on the body.

Lastly, its carotenoids are good for the body but especially great for the heart. Lutein may help prevent heart disease and health problems like atherosclerosis (clogging of arteries) due to its anti-inflammatory properties. Lutein can be found in all greens, broccoli, and even oranges, so you can keep it in your diet year round with no problem.

LEMONGRASS

We know lemongrass as a seasoning we use when cooking, and it is mainly used in Asian cuisine, but did you know lemongrass has over twenty health benefits for the body and can be turned into oil? Interesting, right? From calming an upset stomach, to decreasing swelling, and even fighting antibiotic resistant infections, lemongrass is phenomenal.

First, what is lemongrass? Is it grass that grows from lemons, or is it just grass? Neither. It is an herb from the grass family native to India and Asia. It's packed with nutrients and vitamins and can convert to oil and even tea. Lemongrass is key for a healthy body, and we'll examine just a few key benefits.

As a natural diuretic, lemongrass helps remove toxins from the body. It will increase urination and aid the kidneys and liver in releasing unwanted waste from the body.

Many people experience edema or excess water retention. Lemongrass can help flush the excess fluid out of the body. It also helps balance cholesterol levels and prevents lipids or fats in the bloodstream due to its anti-hyperlipidemic properties. When lemongrass is made into a tea, it can relax the mind and body, aiding in REM sleep and preventing insomnia.

I previously mentioned that lemongrass fights an antibiotic-resistant infection. "Lemongrass essential oil has an anti-biofilm capacity and is beneficial against the infection caused by Staphylococcus aureus.[118] It contains phenols and essential oil, which may disrupt the growth of infections and germs and help inhibit the formation of the biofilms."[119]

Do you suffer from upset stomach, constipation, or ulcerative colitis? Lemongrass can help ease pain and discomfort, reduce inflammation, and improve overall digestion and absorption in the stomach.

Hate springtime because of a constant runny nose, severe cough, puffy eyes, or even fever? Lemongrass is often referred to as the "fever grass" because it induces sweating, therefore helping to reduce the overall body temperature and fever. Also, it is packed with vitamin C to strengthen the immune system and fight against that cold, oxidative stress, and severe cough.

Lemongrass has antifungal and antimicrobial properties to help ward against sores, skin irritations, and yeast infections. My mom once suffered from vertigo, a sensation of whirling and loss of balance, caused by a disease affecting the inner ear or the vestibular nerve.[120] Lemongrass is used to relieve stress or anxiety in the mind. It calms the mind and nerves, relaxing the nervous system, therefore reducing the effects of vertigo.

Do you have acne-prone skin or dark marks like me? Lemongrass is considered an astringent and tonic, which will not only exfoliate the skin but also sterilize, cleanse, and strengthen it.

Lastly, lemongrass helps with weight loss by promoting the use of stored fat as energy for healthy metabolism. So instead of thinking of lemongrass only for culinary purposes, view it as an essential herb for everyday life.

LAVENDER

Lavender is a flower to most, but for some, it is used in the oil form. Lavender oil is the most used essential oil in the world. Its original name is Lavandula stoechas, and it has antimicrobial, antifungal, anti-depressive, and calming effects to help improve our mood.[121]

From healing cuts, moisturizing the hair, aiding in cognitive function, and providing a nice aroma, lavender is a versatile and beneficial essential oil.[122]

We have been told that aloe vera is best at healing cuts, burns, or small lacerations; however, due to lavender's antimicrobial properties, it may help with healing and fight against infection while promoting the production of collagen to repair the skin.[123]

My skin is very sensitive and may react to a subtle change in my diet, perfume, or even lotion. Thankfully, lavender contains antioxidant properties to help fight against oxidative stress and free radical damage while reducing inflammation and redness caused by an allergic reaction.[124] One study showed that lavender can inhibit immediate-type allergic reactions by inhibition of mass cell degranulation. Lavender oil can increase the antioxidants in the body to help naturally fight against toxins and unwanted pathogens from the environment.[125]

Do you struggle to remember minor things? Do you know someone who is currently suffering from Alzheimer's, or do you have a family history of the disease? Lavender oil may improve cognition impairment from Alzheimer's disease. A study conducted at the National Institute of Health showed, "Lavender oil, with the active component linalool, protected the oxidative stress, activity of cholinergic function and expression of proteins of Nrf2/HO-1 pathway, and synaptic plasticity."[126] Therefore, lavender may have neuroprotective effects on the brain.[127]

Migraines—everyone hates them. You may feel like there is no relief, so you keep taking Advil or another pain killer. Lavender essential oil, however, is considered a sedative due to its anti-anxiety and calming effects. Some individuals who suffer from migraines were asked to use lavender oil as a treatment, and the results showed a significant reduction in the migraines, therefore suggesting that inhalation of lavender essential oil may be an effective and safe treatment modality in acute management of migraine headaches.[128] On the other hand, the calming effect of lavender oil is also beneficial to people who struggle to get enough sleep.[129]

During a study of two groups of postpartum women who struggle to sleep, one group used lavender oil as a treatment to improve sleep quality and the other did not. The results showed, "Comparing sleep quality between control and intervention groups after eight weeks from the beginning of the intervention indicated that aromatherapy was effective in the improvement of mothers' sleep quality."[130]

When we experience pain, whether it's a headache, heartache, or pain in our joints, back or menstrual cramps, all we want is relief! Lavender oil may reduce or rid pain in the body. Due to its anti-inflammatory properties and calming effects, it has been known to reduce the pain associated with perineal discomfort following normal childbirth and used as treatment for recurrent aphthous ulceration. It is also able to reduce the pain intensity of needle insertion.

Postpartum depression is often overlooked, yet it is very real, and many women experience it. Just like any other form of depression, it can take over your life and cause you to lose your willingness to live. Lavender essential oil can help. A pilot study was performed on postpartum women to determine the effect lavender oil had on them. The study indicated "positive findings with minimal risk for the use of aromatherapy as a complementary therapy in both anxiety and depression scales with postpartum women."[131]

This essential oil reduces anxiety, relives stress, and improves sleep without side effects unlike its unnatural counterparts. So when looking for pain relief or a mood enhancer, get a diffuser or use even just a few drops of the oil topically, and relief will be around the corner.

LADY'S MANTLE

It may seem this is only for ladies and helping us during our times of need; however, lady's mantle is beneficial for everyone. It's a water-repellent plant that is grown in the summer, and it's traditionally used as a tea throughout the year. Not only does this plant aid in uterus relief during that time of the month, but it also helps the liver, digestive system, and blood pressure. Let's dig a little deeper to see how this plant can benefit us long-term.

Do you have severe menstrual cramps? Lady's mantle has been known to reduce the pain caused by period cramps because the plant contains properties that can relax the blood vessel walls in the body, reducing tension and pain. It not only reduces tension in the uterine walls but throughout the body, possibly aiding to reduce high blood pressure.

Did you know lady's mantle is a natural diuretic that relieves excess water from the body, whether it be from the ankles or all over, and it is a tonic and an astringent? Have a bad stomachache or can't stop going to the restroom? Tannins are known to have anti-diarrheal properties, which means they can stop constant diarrhea, and plants that contain tannins can be taken to relive the pain.[132] Lady's mantle is one of those plants and can be used to dry up the watery secretion.

On another note, lady's mantle has antiviral properties and can help fight against unwanted pathogens and even be used as a gargle to relive a sore throat.[133]

From menstrual pain, to diarrhea, and even coughs and sore throat, lady's mantle can help in numerous ways. Get it in a tea at your favorite farmers market or grocery store and start relieving yourself of pain.

LUNGWORT

What is a lungwort, and what does it do? Well, it does exactly what it sounds like; it helps protect and heal the lungs. Lungwort is a plant native to coastal regions that has been used to heal severe coughs, bronchitis, and other lung ailments. This plant is beneficial due to its antioxidant properties and great at fighting free radical damage. According to globalhealingcenter.com, "Lungwort is effective against harmful organisms that affect lung and chest function due to its high level of flavonoid glycosides, another name for specific types of antioxidants."[134]

Lastly, this plant may help reduce inflammation, aid in asthma treatment, and detoxify the lungs and body. It can be found in the tea isle of your local grocery store or in pill or capsule form at a health food store.

LICORICE ROOT

Licorice root is the root of the glycyrrhiza glabra plant. Native to Europe and Asia, licorice is commonly used in candies but also can be used for medicinal purposes. It can be an excellent aid in reducing the appearance of eczema, and many physicians recommend it in topical skin creams. Licorice root may help with stomach ulcers, improve the lining of the stomach, and repair gut balance because it contains glycyrrhizin acid properties, which have been shown to improve inflammation.

Licorice root has antibacterial properties, making it ideal for plaque along the gum line and tooth decay. Suffer from a bad cough or phlegm? Did you know licorice root helps stimulate phlegm production? But it is the healthy phlegm, aiding in the removal of unwanted bad phlegm, therefore allowing you to breathe freely and without a cough.

We have all heard that our cortisol levels need to be in check to keep from gaining unwanted weight. Licorice root helps promote good cortisol levels by stimulating the adrenal gland, which manages our stress levels. Licorice may come in the liquid form, tea, or even as a powder. Remember, it's not just used for candy!

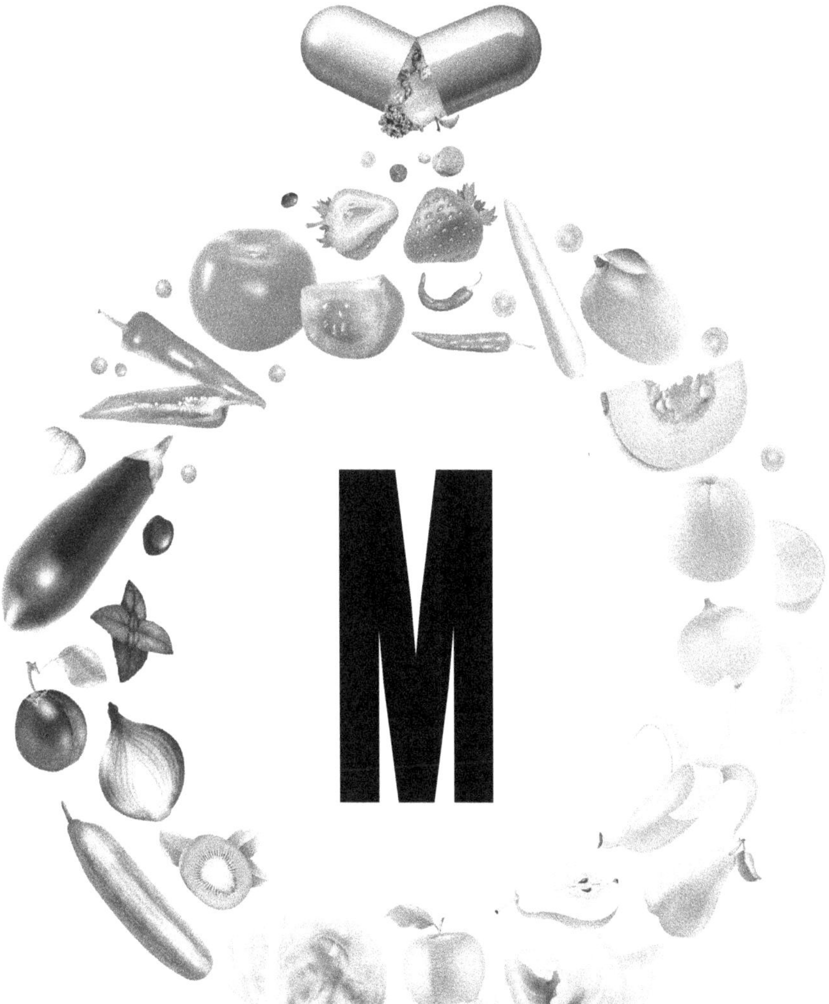
M

MANGO

Some people cannot stand mangoes, claiming they're too slimy and have a tangy taste. But did you know mangoes are considered a mix between a pineapple and a peach? These fruits are not just slimy, they're also very nutrient dense and packed with vitamins and antioxidants. Native to Malaysia and Asia, mangoes range in their benefits, and we will examine how.

Mangoes are high in vitamin C, vitamin A, potassium, and magnesium. These nutrients are important when it comes to regulating blood pressure while providing a low-sodium, juicy snack. They are great at keeping your heart healthy because they contain pectin, and it helps lower cholesterol. Vitamin A is used in a lot of topical creams and serums to keep our skin looking young and youthful. This nutrient is known to decrease wrinkles and promote healthy tissues and tissue repair. Packed with vitamin C, mangoes help build the immune system to fight off infections and protect against oxidative stress and damage.

Do you ever experience a mental fog or forget why you went into a room? Me, too! Vitamin B6 is known for assisting with brain function and improving mental cognition. And you guessed it—Mangoes are full of B vitamins. They're also rich in fiber and low in sugar, helping to balance blood sugar levels. Fiber moves through your system without being digested, causing sugar to be slowly absorbed, leading to balanced sugar levels. The older we get, typically, the weaker our bones and joints get. However, we can combat that with vitamin K and calcium. Mangoes contain a lot of vitamin K in just one cup, providing bone and bone tissue metabolism. Vitamin K works with calcium to maintain strong bones, counteracting bone degradation.

Lastly, the fiber mangoes contain can improve digestive health and prevent constipation by keeping things moving in your system, decreasing your chances of developing gastrointestinal diseases.

MULBERRY

They resemble blackberries and are beneficial to the heart and liver, but they're sweet like figs. Most importantly, mulberries may fight off cancer. They are full of antioxidants that fight free radical damage and protect our cells.

Mulberries contain pectin, which is good for maintaining balanced cholesterol levels. Furthermore, according to the *Journal of Food,* "Science found that the compounds in mulberries helped prevent the oxidation of LDL cholesterol."[135] These berries are low in fat, calories, and sugar, making them ideal for a snack, even aiding in weight loss.

Packed with fiber, they will keep you feeling fuller longer, therefore preventing overeating and helping to maintain a balanced diet and digestive health. They not only are good for digestive health, but also may help with diabetes. With diabetes, it is important to maintain balanced blood sugar levels, and the fiber mulberries have help slow the absorption of sugar into the bloodstream. So mulberries help prevent sugar spikes and keep those levels under control.

Finally, mulberries may help preserve a healthy liver. The liver's role is to remove toxins from the body, break down fats, and clot blood. However, that can be hindered by one's lifestyle and diet. Mulberries contain properties and compounds that help prevent fat accumulation on the liver and aid in the removal of unwanted toxins.[136]

Remember, even though it resembles a blackberry, this little fruit has its own powerful benefits.

MILK THISTLE

Oh, so this is just compressed milk, right? Wrong. Milk thistle is actually an herb that is used to detoxify the liver and body. It helps fight inflammation and increase enzyme formation while improving bile production. Milk thistle has a reputation for fighting liver damage and gallbladder problems.

This herb is native to California but can be grown in other warm areas. It helps fight against free radical damage and oxidative stress while improving the liver's detoxification and filtering unwanted toxins from the environment and our lifestyle. Did you know the liver is a blood filter? That means the liver cleans the blood naturally to remove toxins in order to distribute it throughout the rest of our bodies and organ systems. "The liver helps remove toxicity and harmful substances from our blood, aids in hormone production, detoxifies the body, and releases glucose into the bloodstream in order to give our body steady energy and releases bile into our small intestine so fat can be absorbed from foods."[137]

Do you suffer from cirrhosis of the liver or gallbladder disease? Milk thistle may help repair liver cells, improve liver function, and increase your ability to fight off diseases. Furthermore, it is packed with antioxidants, particularly silymarin, which helps fight against cancer. Silymarin fights cell mutation and damage by stopping the fastening of toxins to the cell membrane. Also, it stops pathogens and toxins from staying in the body, protects healthy cells, and encourages protein synthesis.[138]

Ever have gallstones or kidney stones? I have heard they're extremely painful. Milk thistle may help prevent them because it aids in detoxification and increases the flow of bile, preventing the cholesterol and bile from binding together.

We learned earlier that milk thistle contains antioxidants and helps eliminate unwanted toxins and free radicals in the body. This helps with the skin as well. Milk thistle can protect against wrinkles, sagging skin, dark spots, etc. because it assists in slowing down the aging process. You can purchase it in powder or pill form or even drink it in a tea. Just consume it somehow to reap the benefits.

MELATONIN

Do you have trouble falling asleep? What about staying asleep or getting into REM sleep? Have you tried sleep aids, teas, or listening to soothing sounds, but nothing works? Try melatonin. It's a natural sleep aid that helps slow the body down to prepare for sleep and allows you to get sound, quality rest. Now I know you're thinking, *Yeah, okay, it will help those average people who struggle a little with sleep deprivation, but mine is severe!* Not to worry; melatonin may improve sleep for individuals who travel often and don't have a set sleep pattern, even people who work the night shift and have to get their rest during the day. I didn't forget about my menopausal women who toss and turn all night, fighting to get good sleep. Melatonin can help you as well.

Now that we've established that melatonin helps with sleep, let's explore how else it benefits the body. It may improve the heart and lower cholesterol levels due to the antioxidant and anti-inflammatory components it contains. Furthermore, it relieves stress because it helps control the body's level of stimulation during the day. When you are stressed, you produce more melatonin during the day and less at nighttime, causing an increase in cortisol, the stress hormone, thereby throwing off your body's natural rhythm. A melatonin supplement will decrease your body's overall anxiety and calm the brain, leading to a relaxed mood.

Did you know light emissions cause your melatonin levels to decrease at night, resulting in a tougher time getting to sleep? Therefore, it's always best to limit screen time when it gets close to bedtime.

Remember, daily exercise and getting some natural vitamin D from the sun helps the body produce a natural circadian rhythm, so you'll know when it's time to sleep.

MANGANESE

You may know that manganese isn't a fruit or vegetable, but what is it? It is a trace mineral that is essential for the body's production of bone density and absorption. It's also vital for the organ system functionality in the body. This mineral can be found in several beans and legumes, sprouted grains, and high-antioxidant fruits and vegetables.

The older we get, the weaker our bones become. This is especially true for women. Manganese can help strengthen bone density and may improve osteoporosis. Also, if you suffer from arthritis pain, manganese's ability to reduce inflammation can help ease the pain and discomfort from arthritis.[139]

Furthermore, it helps regulate the hormones and balance iron levels by increasing the absorption rate and usage of iron. On the other hand, manganese helps turn compounds found in food into nutrients the body can use and provides energy within the body as well as amino acids. Manganese can fight inflammation and assist in reducing oxidative stress on the body. Therefore, when it comes to diseases such as Asthma, COPD, and other respiratory issues, manganese may help improve overall lung function.[140]

Lastly, if you're anemic, manganese is especially beneficial for you since it helps with the absorption of iron in the body. Just remember, manganese-rich foods are those beans and legumes we love.

BABY BLUES

My sister gained a good amount of weight after her first child and struggled to get it off. When she became pregnant with my youngest nephew, she said she wanted to do her pregnancy differently this time around. I informed her that the foods she eats while the baby is in the womb affects the baby's weight and appetite for the rest of his life! She was appalled because her physician didn't tell her that. When she went into action, she wanted a low-sugar, high-protein, moderate-fat diet for her pregnancy, not only for herself but for the baby. She had late-night cravings for sweets and didn't know how to cope. She never liked the texture of yogurt, as a lot of people don't; it's an acquired taste. I told her to "doctor it up." She added fresh blueberries, cinnamon, a packet of stevia, and one-fourth cup of granola. She loved it! Not only did it help with her cravings, but she was also getting lots of protein and building the baby's immune system to tolerate dairy. Adding this yogurt treat to her regimen allowed her to resist the sweet temptations and have a healthy baby boy. And she not only lost the baby weight from her first child, but she was back to her high school weight! Making small changes temporarily can have long-lasting results, not just for you, but for your child as well.

N

NEEM OIL

Clearly, we know it is an oil, but where does it come from? Neem oil comes from the neem tree seeds. It is full of antioxidants and serves as a natural pesticide, mosquito repellent, skin moisturizer, and it's even used in beauty products. Neem helps fight oxidative damage caused by free radicals, especially on the skin. Neem oil is considered a pesticide because it contains azadirachtin, a compound that "has a very complex structure, being a mixture of related substances extracted from the neem seed kernels. The seeds are the only source of azadirachtin. Azadirachtin affects insects in many different ways, including acting as an insect growth regulator, anti-feedant, repellent, sterilant and oviposition inhibitor."[141]

Lastly, neem oil may be helpful in moisturizing the skin and keeping a youthful glow because it contains numerous essential fatty acids and vitamin E that can infiltrate the skin. Did you know, commonly, when we apply oil to the skin, the skin begins to shine or get greasy? However, this doesn't happen with neem oil because the vitamin E helps block the oxidization in the skin, resulting in rapid wound healing and vibrant, almost wrinkle-free skin.

When purchasing neem oil, be sure not to get the fragmented or conventionally modified version, but 100 percent pure neem oil.

NUTMEG

It is used in lots of holiday dishes, especially around Thanksgiving and Christmas. I love putting it on my oatmeal, and it even has a pleasant aroma to lighten up a room. Nutmeg tastes great and provides a lot of flavor to food, but did you know nutmeg also has several health benefits for the body? Let's do a little digging and see what we can find.

First, nutmeg may help calm your mood and even be an excellent sleep aid, promoting quality, sound sleep. Maybe Mom knew what she was doing when she gave you that warm milk with a little nutmeg late at night. Furthermore, nutmeg may be good for the heart, helping to reduce "bad" cholesterol and ease the pumping of blood through the body.[142]

Finally, nutmeg is great for the gut and digestion due to the anti-inflammatory compounds found in the seed. Whether you have a large family to cook for, need a good night's rest, or just want to have a good bowel movement, nutmeg can aid you.

NECTARINES

They are similar in appearance to peaches but not fuzzy. I adore them grilled, especially in the summer. There are different types, from white to yellow and even red. Did you know the different color nectarines provide different nutrients and vitamins? But all of them are packed with antioxidants to fight off free radical damage, and they're high in fiber and low in sugar.

Let's start with fiber. As Americans, we never get enough, as most of our foods are processed and high in sugar. However, nectarines are full of fiber, making you feel fuller longer and adding bulk to your stool to keep things moving through the gastrointestinal system. Furthermore, high-fiber foods can aid in weight loss because the body processes them slowly and they help prevent sugar cravings, causing us to eat less throughout the day. Less sugar cravings help to prevent diabetes and balance our sugar levels.

Nectarines are also good at increasing absorption in the body due to the prebiotic effect it has on the stomach and gut. It helps the body maintain good gut bacteria, causing a decreased chance to develop sickness. They contain lots of vitamin C, which strengthen the immune system and fights off unwanted germs and illnesses, keeping us healthy.

Is macular degeneration or cataracts something that runs in your family? It doesn't run in mine, but I just found out that glaucoma does. Well, nectarines can help improve vision and might help decrease the risk of developing macular degeneration and cataracts because they are full of vitamin A. Vitamin A is crucial when it comes to eye health and preventing disease.

On another note, nectarines contain two compounds out of the several we consume daily that may improve overall eye health. According to an article by the National Institute of Health, "Of the 40 to 50 carotenoids typically consumed in the human diet, lutein and zeaxanthin are deposited at and up to five fold higher content in the macular region of the retina."[143] This means it helps to decrease vision loss.

Nectarines are great for the heart in numerous ways. First, they are packed with potassium, which may lower blood pressure and help with certain diseases of the heart. Also, since they are fiber and nutrient rich, the cholesterol levels stay balanced and help lower triglyceride levels. They contain plant polyphenols, which are antioxidants that may help ward off diseases, treat digestion issues, help prevent heart disease, and assist with weight management. Even though they look like peaches, remember, nectarines don't have the fuzz, but they can make a lot of good fuss in the body.

NIACIN

Niacin, commonly known as vitamin B3, is a water-soluble vitamin that is essential for the body in all organ systems, especially when it comes to the transfer of food to energy for use in the body. From the heart, to the brain, the stomach and even the skin, niacin is needed in more ways than one. Vegetarians and vegans must make sure they are taking their vitamins daily because, without them, they lose all the nutrients we get from animals. Niacin is primarily found in large quantities in poultry and fish. It's also in avocado and sweet potato, but over eighty percent of the recommended daily allowance (RDA) comes from one serving of chicken.

Dementia is a common disorder within the elderly population; however, niacin is beneficial for the brain and helps with memory, and it promotes good cognition and less brain fog. It helps the brain by activating the synapses to think and use energy to connect. Niacin is great for the heart because it helps fight inflammation, one of the many problems related to heart disease. It also reduces oxidative stress and promotes balanced cholesterol levels. Do you suffer from sore joints or pain, or have you been diagnosed with arthritis? Niacin can help improve your symptoms due to its ability to fight against chronic inflammation and stiffness, aiding in increased mobility of the joints and reduced pain.

Finally, let's look at the skin. Do you have eczema or acute dermatitis? Is your skin always dry, itching, and scaly? If so, it may be a sign of a vitamin B3 or niacin deficiency. Increasing your intake of niacin-rich foods such as chicken, tuna, or peanuts, may bring you some relief. So before trying niacin in the pill form, remember, it's always better to get your vitamins through food if and when possible.

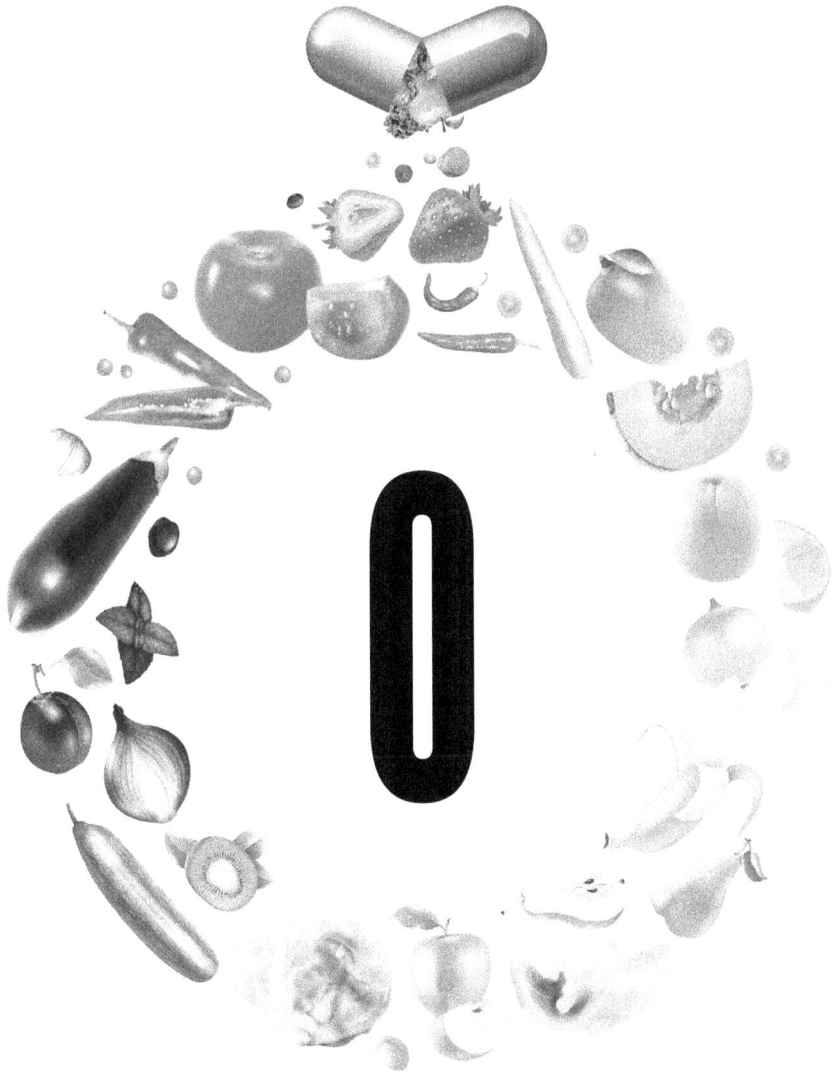

OLIVE LEAF

Olive leaf extract comes from the olive leaf tree native to Africa and Asia. Olive leaf contains several different compounds, but one in particular, oleuropein, is known for its health benefits such as being an antiviral and antibacterial compound. Olive leaf has been used for many years for medicinal purposes and now is even used as a tea. We are going to explore some of the health benefits and why this should be a staple in our diets.

Olive leaf has been known to help lower blood pressure and reduce the LDL cholesterol when taken consistently over a period of time, according to a study done by the National Health Institute.[144]

Do you have high cholesterol or are you always worried about what foods you should eat to prevent high cholesterol? Olive leaf extract may help improve your overall cholesterol levels and decrease chronic inflammation that's typically associated with it. It can help improve overall heart health and reduce stress on the heart.

Prediabetic or type 2 diabetic? Olive leaf extract can also aid with diabetes. "Olive leaf extracts have hyperglycemic effects, meaning they reduce blood sugar levels in the body. The olive leaf also controls blood glucose levels in the body. The polyphenols in olive leaf play a vital role in delaying the production of sugar."[145] Diabetes runs big in my family, so once I learned this, I was intrigued and purchased some olive leaf. Diabetes can be improved by making small changes in your daily life and diet.

Olive leaf extract also helps with osteoarthritis, which is caused by the joints and bones rubbing together due to a reduction of cartilage between them. However, since olive leaf is an anti-inflammatory, it can be considered a natural aid because it reduces the amount of inflammation present in the joints, causing less pain and more comfort and cushion.

On a lighter note, did you know olive leaf is good for the skin? Its antioxidants help protect healthy skin cells while preventing damage and oxidation. It can help you maintain beautiful skin and even improve the skin's firmness and elasticity.

Remember, I mentioned that olive leaf extract has antiviral properties. It has been known to fight off infections, viruses, and the common cold. Olive leaf extract combats certain microbes, prevents the replication of the viruses, and destroys unwanted pathogens, causing a lower chance of sickness. From UTI's to candida and even fatigue, olive leaf extract fights off infections and illnesses. According to a study done in 2003 at the National Institute of Health, olive leaf extract was able to kill off bacteria from genital infections, skin infections, and even the intestines. Olive leaf acts as a natural antibiotic, combating bacteria and fungus because of its antimicrobial effect.[146]

Suffer from brain fog or even something as severe as dementia and you want some relief? Olive leaf may improve brain function and combat memory loss. The oleuropein it contains is known to improve brain health and reduce signs of dementia and degradation of brain function. It fights against the oxidative stress and damage that normally would occur in the brain and helps maintain healthy brain cells.

Olive leaf can provide you with more energy, less joint and muscle pain, and it even helps repair and heal cuts and bruises. You can purchase it at your local grocery store; just make sure it is organic.

ORANGES

Thought to be the number-one source of vitamin C, from Cuties to clementine and more, this fruit is packed with antioxidants and fiber, and they're low in sugar. Oranges help with inflammation and weight loss. They also boost your immune system and much more. We know they're full of antioxidants, which are known to fight against free radical damage and help prevent added stress on the body. But oranges also help build your resistance to illness and infection. They have been proven to shorten the duration of a cold and help prevent the reoccurrence of sickness due to the high amount of vitamin C they contain.[147]

Did you know some oranges contain blood? I'm kidding; however, there are blood oranges. These oranges are slightly sweeter than the traditional orange, and they have a deep red, almost purple interior. Blood oranges get their color from anthocyanins, which is a type of flavonoid that gives a lot of fruits and vegetables their pigment. When I was in school studying nutrition, I learned a lot about the gut and how it is important to keep it healthy because it can determine whether you develop diseases. Oranges are an excellent choice for a fiber source because they are low in calories and packed with fiber. They will keep you fuller longer, aiding in less consumption of unwanted snacks and foods and help push stool through the digestive system, which is great for individuals who suffer from frequent constipation. Also, they aid the good bacteria you already have in your gut since they act as a prebiotic.

Have you ever wondered why most facial scrubs or masks contain some form of citrus? Oranges can fight off and maybe reverse sun damage and act as an anti-aging treatment. Also, when you apply the peel of an orange to the skin, it helps exfoliate and moisturize. Oranges can provide a protective layer to the skin when eaten regularly and help achieve that radiant glow we all desire by drying out acne.

Oranges have been shown to improve the heart and aid in maintaining good cognitive function. According to studies from the National Library of Medicine, "Citrus fruit can help protect against heart disease, and the more intake of citrus fruit, better performance in several cognitive abilities was found."[148]

From small oranges to large ones and even blood oranges, citrus fruit can help us in ways we've never thought of. This doesn't mean you should just go out and buy orange juice. Remember to eat your calories; don't drink them. The actual fruit has *way* more benefits than the sugar-packed juices we see in the store.

OATS

Oats are a staple for the elderly, but it is known to lower cholesterol, too. Let's examine how oats are beneficial. If you are vegetarian or vegan, oats are a good choice for consumption. In less than a one-cup serving, they contain more than seven grams of protein and provide great nutrients and antioxidants. Oats are always recommended from your doctor as a good source of fiber, and it's great for lowering cholesterol, but how? They contain a fiber called beta-glucans, which are polysaccharides, a fiber that lowers cholesterol. According to an article published by the National Institute of Health, "Intake of oat β-glucan at daily doses of at least 3g may reduce plasma total and low-density lipoprotein (LDL) cholesterol levels by 5-10% in normo-cholesterolemic or hyper-cholesterolemic subjects."[149]

Therefore, people who are at risk for high cholesterol or already have it can truly benefit from eating oats. Also, beta-glucans fight against excessive inflammation in the body, which is known to be the root cause of most diseases, and it builds up our immune system to fight off infections and illnesses.

Oats are great for breakfast because they can help maintain balanced sugar levels throughout the day and keep you fuller longer due to the high fiber content. Oat bran is actually where all the fiber is contained, and when shopping for oats, rolled oats are best because the oat bran is still intact, versus quick oats. With such a high fiber content, not only will you be full, your digestive system will maintain regularity, and you may even lose weight. Furthermore, the oats will remove unwanted toxins from your system and help prevent issues such as colon cancer or other digestive problems because you will be able to preserve a healthy gut and overall body system.

Lastly, oats are great for individuals who are at risk for osteoporosis or osteopenia. *How so?* Oats contain phosphorus and manganese, which are both essential for bone health. These minerals are not only crucial for the enzymatic production of bones but also maintaining healthy bones and protecting them from decay. Whether you are making oatmeal cookies, traditional oatmeal with blueberries, which is how I like it, or using oats as a topping on a pie, remember to choose rolled oats and enjoy every bite!

OAKMOSS

Are we referring to something similar to oatmeal? Not quite. Oakmoss is an essential oil. Like most essential oils, it can help with the skin and provide soothing effects to the mood. Furthermore, it has the ability to help rid unwanted bacteria from the skin due to its antiseptic properties. You can even apply it to irritated skin or eczema to help relieve itching. From a skin smoother to a mood calmer, oakmoss is helpful for the mind and body. Just make sure you get 100 percent pure oakmoss essential oil to reap the benefits.

ONION

They come red, yellow, and white. They can be eaten raw or cooked. They have a strong aroma and taste great on burgers. Onions, surprisingly, are packed with health benefits for us, so let's dig in. Onions are full of antioxidants, particularly flavonoids, and can help fight against inflammation and a lot of common diseases, and they even help with sickness. One of the most important flavonoids they contain are ACSOs. ACSO stands for "alkenyl cysteine sulfoxides," which impart a red/purple color to some onion varieties. The ACSOs are the flavor precursors, which, when cleaved by the enzyme alliinase, generate the characteristic odor and taste of onion. According to the National Library of Medicine, onions have been reported to have "anticarcinogenic properties, antiplatelet activity, antithrombotic activity, anti-asthmatic, and antibiotic effects."[150]

Onions also help fight cancer, from digestive cancers, mouth cancer, and other organs, due to the high antioxidant properties and sulfur they hold. They may also help combat cancer replication.[151]

When we have a cold, we usually reach for lemon or another citrus fruit; however, you may want to grab an onion the next time you're ill. They have been known to fight against respiratory infections, open your sinuses, and rapidly rid the body of excess mucus. On the other hand, onions can help improve heart function while lowering LDL cholesterol. They help fight against free radical damage and reduce inflammation, which improves blood movement and circulation throughout the heart and body and decreases unwanted stress. Additionally, onions contain chromium, which has been known to balance blood sugar and possibly combat and decrease your chances of developing diabetes.

Women, as we get older, we typically have a higher risk for bone fractures and breakage than men. Therefore, maintaining our bone density the older we get is crucial. Onions may help improve bone density and decrease fractures because they contain enzymatic substances, gamma-L-glutamyl-trans-S-1-propenyl-L-cysteine sulfoxides, which are known to prevent osteoporosis and bone decay.[152]

Ever wonder why we cry when slicing an onion? Cutting the onion releases enzymes because we're breaking the cellular membranes that contain the ACSOs. Just splash some lemon juice on the onion prior to cutting, and it should help relieve the discomfort. From fertility to arthritis and their delicious taste, onions help us in more ways than I knew. I will be adding more to my diet.

OIL OF OREGANO

Commonly overlooked and rarely thought of as a healer. Oil of oregano is an herb but used as an essential oil for great health benefits. It has antibacterial, antiviral, and antibiotic properties that positively affect the body. Unlike traditional antibiotics, it's not harmful and can not only heal your body internally, but it also helps treat fungus and bacteria on the skin. Oil of oregano is also like a traditional antibiotic in ways. How, you ask? The medicinal form of oil of oregano contains carvacrol, which is a phenol compound that fights bacteria without killing the healthy bacteria we need.[153]

According to a study from the National Institute of Health, "Carvacrol has merged for its wide spectrum activity extended to food spoilage or pathogenic fungi, yeast and bacteria as well as human, animal and plant pathogenic microorganisms including drug-resistant and biofilm forming microorganisms."[154] That means oil of oregano can fight even drug-resistant strands of organisms and fight yeast and fungi.

You will not have any side effects or harm your immune system with oil of oregano. It's helpful in fighting unnecessary inflammation because the antioxidant properties it has can assist in combating oxidative stress and free radical damage. Most diseases we face, like IBD, arthritis, etc., are due to chronic inflammation, and they can possibly be alleviated with the assistance of oil of oregano.

Thymol is one of the main phenols in oil of oregano because it is an antifungal, helping to rid fungi and prevent further replication. From an upset stomach to food poisoning, a yeast infection, and even athlete's foot, oil of oregano can aid you and provide relief due to the compounds it contains. Remember to purchase the medicinal grade of 100 percent oil of oregano.

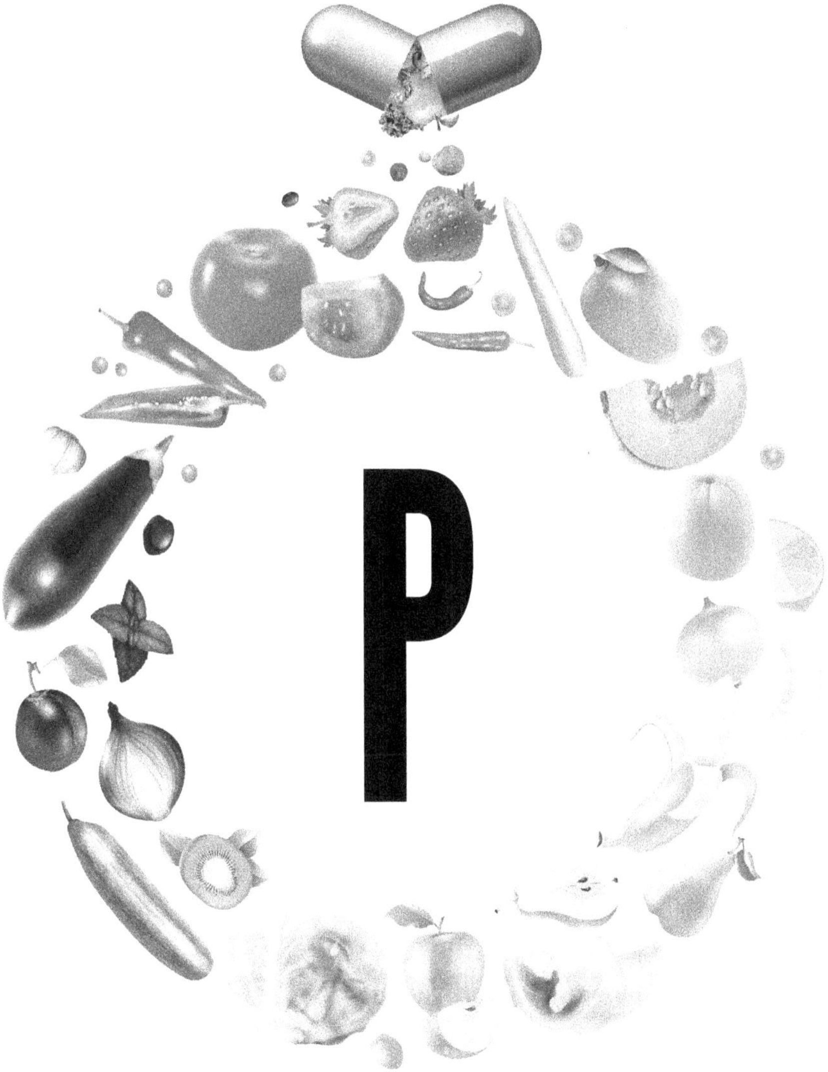
P

PINEAPPLE

These bad boys are great grilled, blended in a smoothie, eaten fresh, or added to your favorite meal for sweetness. One of my favorite things about pineapples is that they fight inflammation and are perfect for that post-workout snack to help reduce the effect of delayed onset muscle soreness or DOMS. This is due to its bromelain, an enzyme known for breaking down proteins into smaller substance-like amino acids in the body. Bromelain also helps slow blood clotting and prevent the formation of clogged blood vessels and arteries, preventing heart attacks and improving overall heart health.

Pineapples are packed with fiber, vitamin C, and calcium. Are you like me and no matter how healthy you feel, you always manage to get sick or catch a cold? Pineapples can provide some relief. The vitamin C content is more than the needed daily amount in just one cup, and we know vitamin C can help fight off infections and illness while strengthening the immune system. Also, vitamin C is great at combating free radical damage and oxidative stress and even helps the skin and nails by acting as an antioxidant in the body to help create collagen and improve cells and organ tissues.

On the other hand, pineapples can help assist in reproduction, but how? Packed with antioxidants, pineapples fight against cell damage, helping to rebuild tissues throughout the body, improve blood flow, and increase sperm count in men. Pineapples also make you "taste good" and give off a pleasant aroma in the genital areas.

Pineapples are excellent for people who suffer from diabetes to help them consume more fiber from whole foods instead of processed foods and for those who want to include more fiber in their diets or reduce the frequency of constipation. This high fiber fruit helps ease digestion and, in turn, may help reduce stomach pain and bloating by quickly helping to remove unwanted waste and toxins from the body.

Do you suffer from arthritis or joint pain? The bromelain in pineapple can assist yet again. "Bromelain works on inflammation by blocking metabolites that cause swelling. It also decreases swelling by activating a chemical in the blood that breaks down fibrin, thus leading to reduced swelling."[155]

Have you ever eaten pineapple and noticed your mood instantly improved? This is due to the amino acid L-tryptophan,[156] which is found only in food, and once ingested, our bodies convert it to serotonin and melatonin. Serotonin levels in the brain determine our mood, and melatonin helps us calm down and improve sleep. Therefore, pineapple can make you happy and help you sleep. Seems like a win-win to me. Make your famous pineapple upside down cake, slice it up and eat it before sexual intercourse, or blend it into your post-workout smoothie. Whichever method you choose, enjoy more pineapples.

PAPAYA

Did you know papaya trees come in male and female form and as a hermaphrodite? Yet the hermaphrodite tree is the only one that produces papaya. Hmm … interesting! Papaya is a fruit native to Mexico and contains the enzyme papain, which helps break down protein into amino acids and peptides, one of the reasons papaya is commonly used when tenderizing meat.[157]

Great, now we know where papaya comes from, but how does it help us? Well, one of its biggest benefits for us is its assistance with digestion and absorption. As Americans, a lot of us eat *way* too much meat and/or protein, and it is hard for our bodies to properly digest it, often leading to constipation. However, papaya can help break down those proteins and prevent constipation and assist with a smooth digestion and release. Also, papaya may help increase the platelet count and strengthen the blood base according to a study on mice conducted by The National Institute of Health: "The group having received palm oil only showed a protracted increase of platelet counts that was significant at hours 8 and 48 and obviously the result of a hitherto unknown stimulation of thrombocyte release. The results call for a dose-response investigation and for extending the studies to the isolation and identification of the C. papaya substances responsible for the release and/or production of thrombocytes."[158]

This means papaya may have the ability to help people who have thrombocytopenia, which is a condition that causes a low blood platelet count.

On the other hand, this tropical fruit contains high levels of vitamin C, which help improve the immune system as well as the heart by fighting against plaque buildup in the arterial walls. Ever wonder where that beautiful rich, deep pigmentation of the papaya comes from? Beta-carotene is a nutrient that not only helps with the rich color but also aids in eye health. Furthermore, certain flavonoids like zeaxanthin aid in combating macular degeneration and harmful rays to the retina. Not only do flavonoids help the eyes but also the skin to protect against oxidative damage that may cause wrinkles and frown lines.[159]

Ever had a ringworm? I know I have, and they are painful. Papaya to the rescue. Its papain fights against infections on the skin by breaking down the proteins and reducing the reproduction or spread of viruses and bacteria. Just remember, you can eat papaya seeds if you choose; they're beneficial just bitter in taste, and this tropical fruit is best eaten when ripe and grown in warm climates.

PEARS

There are more than 1000 varieties of pears. They are low in calories but full of nutrients. From red to green, a soft exterior to a tougher one, pears are bursting with fiber, vitamin C, vitamin A, vitamin E, and folate. However, one of the top health benefits pears offers us is vitamin K. Vitamin K is needed to maintain strong bones. It's better for our skeletal system than calcium. Osteoporosis, arthritis, and osteopenia are all conditions for which pears can provide relief because of their vitamin K and boron. *What's boron?* Boron is a mineral used for building strong bones and muscles and increasing testosterone levels while improving thinking skills and muscle coordination.[160]

Pears are a great substitute for when those sweet cravings hit because they're low in sugar, which is great for diabetic individuals and can be used to give you a boost of energy prior to an intense workout. Pears of all varieties are full of fiber, so if you've ever experienced hemorrhoids, pears are your friend. The high fiber allows stool to move freely through your body while fighting against oxidative stress and inflammation of the colon. Pears, like most fruit, contain pectin, which is a starch that binds or holds together to trap liquid, making it a natural diuretic that eases our digestive system so it can move stool freely. The high amount of fiber pears have will help you feel fuller longer, resulting in a decreased appetite and weight loss.

If pectin can provide such benefits for digestion, what else can it do? Pectin is great for the heart as well, helping to lower cholesterol because it may help free up the arterial wall that could have plaque buildup.

Lastly, pears are full of vitamin C, which provides benefits to us in a number of ways. Vitamin C helps our immune system fight against infections and illness. It keeps our metabolism moving and aids in repairing cells and tissues in the body. Also, it protects our skin from sun damage and combats cell mutation and growth. Pears contain other antioxidants and phenols that provide benefits, but glutathione, particularly, fights against several diseases, from hypertension, cancer, coronary artery disease, and even diverticulosis.

From Anju to bosc and the common Bartlett pear, be sure to eat the skin because that's where a lot of the pear's benefits and nutrients lie.

PALM OIL

Are we referring to oil that comes from palm trees or an oil you can put into your palms to reap the benefits? Neither. Palm oil comes from the fruit of the tree—oil palms. The highest quality of palm oil comes from a tree native to Southwest Africa. Palm oil is packed with antioxidants, may help lower cholesterol, and contains phenols and flavonoids as well as many vitamins and nutrients to provide us with optimal health.

Let's first dive into cholesterol. *Wait, this is oil; isn't that bad for your cholesterol?* Yes and no, depending on the type of oil you consume, it can affect your body and arteries positively or negatively. In this instance, palm oil is great for your heart and the arterial walls. According to a study comparing oils' effect on the cholesterol, "Compared with entry values, the PA (palm oil) diet caused significant reductions in serum total cholesterol, LDL-cholesterol and total Cholesterol/HDL-Cholesterol during the first 6 wk and also a significant reduction in TC/HDL-C during the second 6 wk."[161]

On the other hand, palm oil may improve cognition and brain function. Palm oil contains tocotrienols, which are a group of compounds in the vitamin E family. They're antioxidants that fight inflammation and support proper brain focus. Also, palm oil has vitamin E, which helps improve the appearance of scars on the surface of the skin and provides a youthful glow.

Do you experience dry eyes, blurry vision, or poor health? Palm oil helps the body absorb vitamin A because it contains a lot of beta-carotene. Vitamin A is essential for maintaining proper vision and strengthening the immune system to fight off free radicals and prevent infections. When you eat foods that are high in antioxidants, they combat free radicals and pathogens, defusing any damage that could have been done to our cells and organ tissues. Don't just think of oil as a negative thing, try to find the best quality oil and/or fats to aid the cholesterol in the body.

PUMPKIN

They're big, orange, round, and everyone picks them in October; however, pumpkins are more than just something people carve for Halloween or bake into their favorite dessert. Pumpkins contain essential nutrients for our body and provide a wide array of benefits. They are high in beta-carotene, which our bodies convert into vitamin A, and we know vitamin A is essential for eye health. They are made up of about ninety percent water, making them low in calories and a great diet food option. On the other hand, pumpkins are rich in fiber and may help with weight-loss by riding the body of unwanted toxins and bacteria.

Pumpkins are loaded with antioxidants that fight free radical damage and help combat damage to our cells. Also, being rich in vitamin C, pumpkins strengthen our immune systems and even help our wounds and cuts heal faster by increasing our white blood cell production and helper T cells.

Wish you had more radiant or youthful skin? Pumpkin is the key! Vitamin C is great for the skin because it helps the body make collagen, which aids in healthy skin cells and prevents wrinkles.

So whether you choose to make pumpkin soup in the winter, use pumpkin as a pasta substitute by spiraling it, or grill it, think of pumpkin as a versatile vegetable, not just something kids carve during Halloween.

PRICKLY PEAR

Sometimes called nopal, prickly pear isn't a pear; it's actually cactus. It's grown in warm climates and, due to its high-water content, it's great for times of drought or if you suffer from dehydration, especially in the summer. Also, this cactus is packed with antioxidants and has anti-inflammatory effects on the body, fighting off disease and boosting the immune system to further prevent illness.[162]

Had a great night out with friends and drank too much? Prickly pear can help with the all-too-common hangover, and the carotenoids it contains help protect the liver and remove harmful toxins from the body. You can boil prickly pear or even make it into your favorite jelly to have on your morning toast.

POTATO (SWEET)

I love them as a breakfast hash or for fries. Sweet potato is unlike any other potato. It's high in antioxidants, contains about four times the recommended daily value of vitamin A, it's packed with vitamin C, and low in fat.

Let's dig into why sweet potato is great for even those watching their waistlines. Sweet potato can provide you with the needed energy to get you through an intense workout because they are slowly absorbed in the body. Furthermore, they're packed with fiber, and they're nutrient dense, keeping you fuller longer, aiding in weight loss because you're not hungry, and it helps curb your sweet cravings.

Suffer from poor eyesight, at risk for macular degeneration, or experience floaters? Vitamin A is essential for maintaining proper eye health and slowing down eye-related diseases. Sweet potatoes contain plenty of vitamin A, making them, without a doubt, the root vegetable of choice to help combat these illnesses. Vitamin A is also important for a healthy and strong immune system. This key vitamin assists T cells in fighting off illness and infections and help prevent the same sickness from occurring again. The richer the color or pigment of food the more antioxidants it contains, hence why purple sweet potatoes contain the highest amount of antioxidants of all potatoes. Granted, sweet potatoes contain a great deal as well. They receive their color from beta-carotene, an antioxidant, and we know antioxidants fight chronic inflammation and combat free radical damage. Ingesting foods high in antioxidants helps decrease your chances of developing common diseases such as autoimmune disorders and even heart disease.

Lastly, sweet potatoes may help balance blood sugar because the high fiber content helps slow the rate at which sugar is absorbed in the blood stream, ultimately helping to prevent spikes and drops. Make a pie, grill it with other veggies, or add it to your morning breakfast routine. Whichever method you choose, just enjoy that potato.

PEPPERMINT

More than just a candy or a leaf, peppermint can provide health benefits when used as an essential oil. From calming your mood and nausea to improving muscle soreness, fighting colds and illness, and boosting energy, it is versatile and effective.[163] Peppermint oil has been dated back to ancient Egyptian times for medicinal purposes, and it is a hybrid of spearmint and water mint. Do you have irritable bowel syndrome? One study revealed that peppermint oil may be effective at relieving the symptoms associated with IBS, and when given as an enema, it can even provide relief to the colon due to its muscle relaxing properties.[164]

Suffer from allergies, frequent sinus infections, or sore throat? Peppermint oil is excellent at riding mucus and opening the nasal cavity because the active components have antibacterial, antioxidant, and antiviral properties, making it ideal to combat respiratory infections and reduce inflammation. Often, when we get sick, we forget about our chest. Applying peppermint oil to our chest can open the airflow and help relieve congestion.

During the summer, many of us enjoy lying out by the pool; however, what we don't like is getting burned by the sun. Peppermint oil can help provide relief from sunburn by helping to heal the skin faster, inhibit itching, and soften and tone the skin.[165]

Furthermore, its antiseptic and anti-inflammatory properties aid in preventing blackheads, eczema, skin infections, and oily skin.[166]

Ever use peppermint oil in your hair? You probably have but didn't know it because it is used in several shampoos and conditioners. Peppermint oil naturally helps rid dandruff and infections that may lie on the scalp with its antiseptic properties. Additionally, it helps repair damaged hair, improve thinning hair, decrease dandruff, and stimulate the scalp and follicle growth. One study showed peppermint oil to be more effective than other more known oils such as jojoba oil and saline. The results suggested that peppermint oil induced a rapid anagen stage and could be used as a practical agent for hair growth.[167]

Are you a mother? Do you have a newborn, or have you been around a newborn that has colic? Colic occurs when healthy babies cry for prolonged periods of time. This is often one of the hardest times for mother and child. Peppermint oil may help. One double-blind study found that peppermint oil provided much relief for babies and their mothers.[168]

Lastly, peppermint oil can be used to freshen breath. The menthol it contains helps fight against infections and bacteria that typically lie on the tongue and gum line, hence why most toothpaste tastes like peppermint.[169]

From improving the hair and energy levels to reducing infections on the skin and in the mouth, peppermint oil can be used in several ways to improve your body and overall health.

POMEGRANATE

It's one of the most difficult fruits to eat. It has a hard shell and small, sweet pebbles inside. Did you know you can get all the pomegranate seeds out by simply soaking the fruit in water for about five minutes then breaking it in half and turning it over and hitting it hard with a wooden spoon on the back? All the seeds will fall out. Genius, I know. Pomegranate seeds aren't just red, juicy pebbles that are nice to look at; they also have health benefits.

Struggle with proper digestion, inflammation, high cholesterol or getting in the mood? Pomegranate seeds help with all of those afflictions. They're also packed with vitamin C and antioxidants to not only give you energy but also help fight against infection. Pomegranates may increase blood flow and the chances for an erection while stimulating testosterone levels in men.[170]

Pomegranate has anti-cancer effects for women and men. According to a study done by the US National Institute of Medicine, "Pomegranate extracts have been used as anti-cancer agents and they contain a large number of potentially bioactive substances. Punicic acid is an omega-5 fatty acid capable of inhibiting breast cancer proliferation and is found in Punica granatum (pomegranate) seed oil."[171]

Pomegranates are good at fighting off infections because of their complex compounds. From flavonoids to anthocyanins and even the punicic acid I just mentioned, pomegranates may improve diarrhea, upset stomach, or ulcers. They also balance gut flora and ward off microbial infections. One of the most under-consumed fruits, pomegranates contain one of the best nutrients for individuals who suffer from high cholesterol or have a family history of heart disease. Did you know that if you drink the juice of pomegranates, you are drinking the highest number of antioxidants for your body than any other fruit juice? Hmm … interesting. Maybe you should opt out of that apple or orange juice and get pomegranate instead. The antioxidants in pomegranate juice may help improve arterial flow and prevent plaque buildup. Pomegranate juice can also help improve blood pressure and the overall function of the heart.[172]

Lastly, they contain flavonoids, which, once inside the body, act as anti-inflammatory instruments, thereby reducing excessive inflammation in the body. Just remember, when eating pomegranates, don't fight with the fruit; just use a wooden spoon to help ease the seeds out.

PINE BARK

Pine bark, like the tree? Yes, pine bark extract is an herbal extract common to the United Kingdom, and it's derived from the Pinus tree. It may help prevent ailments from osteoarthritis to high blood pressure. It can increase exercise stamina and even help boost sexual drive, all due to the antioxidant compounds, oligomeric proanthocyanin, they contain.

Pine bark extract can improve many health conditions because it also gives off anti-inflammatory, antibacterial, and antiviral properties that help fight off infections and many common diseases. One of the main reasons I was interested in learning more about pine bark extract was because it helps with hyperpigmentation and protecting the body against sun damage. According to one study, pine bark not only provides photoprotection, but may be used to reduce hyperpigmentation of human skin and improve skin barrier function and extracellular matrix homeostasis.[173]

Pine bark extract also reduces chronic inflammation because it fights against free radical damage and ultimately increases immune health. Are you a competitive athlete who is worried about your reaction time or just someone trying to improve your workouts? Pine bark was used in a study to see the effects it had on athletic performance, and the study demonstrated that pine bark improves fatigue by increasing the serum NAD$^+$ levels.[174] In a recent study, it showed that an acute single dose of pine bark supplement improved endurance performance in trained athletes.[175]

Lastly, due to its abundance of antioxidants, pine bark may improve blood glucose levels and fight off infections and bacteria while improving our hearing and boosting our immune systems. You can purchase pine bark extract at your local health food store in the pill or tablet form.

PASSIONFLOWER

Not only beautiful in appearance but also plentiful in health benefits, passionflower is more than just a flower; it's a plant that fights inflammation, skin rashes or eczema, and even high blood pressure—just to name a few. Sometimes used in calming tea or extracts, passionflower can help with anxiety and depression because it helps increase GABA levels in the brain. GABA is gamma-aminobutyric acid that sends chemical messages through the brain and the nervous system and is involved in regulating communication between brain cells.[176] Passionflower helps fight against menopausal symptoms like hot flashes and night sweats.[177]

Suffer from insomnia or high sugar levels? Passionflower may help improve sleep by calming the cells in the body and turning off the brain at night. Also, it helps balance blood sugar levels and fights excessive inflammation due to the antioxidant and phytonutrient properties it contains.

When I get overwhelmed, my anxiety spikes, and I know I'm not alone. Passionflower can help us because it provokes a calm and relaxed mood over the body due to its ability to increase the GABA (mood receptors) in our brains. When I'm anxious, my blood pressure rises, but passionflower helps reduce my systolic blood pressure and gets my numbers back in range.

So from menopause, to sugar levels, depression, blood pressure, and sleep, passionflower and its components can help bring comfort and relief.

PARSLEY

I don't know how many times I have mistaken this herb for cilantro. Did you know parsley has so many health benefits that some people consider it a superfood? Crazy, I know. Parsley has antibacterial, antifungal, and antioxidant properties, just to mention a few. However, the health benefits of parsley are plentiful, so bear with me as I break it down for you.

First, parsley is packed with antioxidants, and this is crucial because antioxidants help fight oxidative stress and free radical damage, which are known as the main culprits for several diseases. Do you suffer from seasonal allergies, asthma, or plaque buildup? Parsley contains vitamins C and A. Vitamin C is important for maintaining a healthy immune system and fighting off and reducing excess inflammation. It also aids in keeping a healthy gut environment. When your immune system is strong, you decrease your chances of catching an illness, and it helps suppress those seasonal allergies. *Well, what about vitamin A?* Parsley's antioxidants and vitamin A are beneficial for eye health. Helping to prevent macular degeneration, glaucoma, and cataracts, parsley can be used to protect the retina and benefit the eye. Furthermore, parsley contains folate, which is responsible for maintaining a healthy heart because it's a B vitamin that helps us convert amino acid in the blood. Also, we know folate is especially important for pregnant women and for the fetus to get proper developmental nutrients.

Do you have bad breath? Even halitosis? Parsley has your back. As a natural antibacterial, it fights and kills bacteria that causes bad breath. It even helps clear up marks, hyperpigmentation, and blemishes on the skin when converted to an oil.

Suffer from frequent constipation or bloated and upset stomach? Parsley is a natural diuretic and helps activate the kidney to excrete excess water from the body and stomach. This helps with edema and provides ease and comfort to the body.[178]

Lastly, parsley may fight the formation of cancer cells. According to a study conducted at the American Association of Cancer, a compound found in parsley called apigenin was examined, and they found that apigenin prevents induced acceleration of tumor development.[179]

Even though parsley is small in size, it is mighty in power and benefits. Remember, if you are going to purchase parsley, smell it first, and don't mistake it for cilantro. If you're picking it up in the oil form, make sure it's a 100-percent pure essential oil.

Parsnip

What are parsnips? Are they just big white carrots? Actually, no. Parsnips are root vegetables that have a high starch content, which make them ideal for making healthier French fries. However, just like carrots, parsnips are great for eye health, but they also provide health benefits for the heart, and they increase regularity of the bowels. The high fiber content makes going to the restroom a breeze, and your stomach will be at ease. Are you a woman with a family history of osteoporosis or osteopenia? Manganese is a key mineral needed to have and maintain strong, healthy bones. Parsnips contain manganese and may help improve bone density and prevent manganese deficiency.

Parsnips contain vitamin C, potassium, and folate along with fiber, which helps improve blood flow and overall heart health. For pregnant women, folate ensures the growing fetus is getting the desired nutrients, and it's essential in helping to prevent birth defects like brain damage or spina bifida.

It's important to understand that folate and folic acid are not the same. Folic acid is commonly added to foods, but folate is a nutrient we need and must get through food or vitamin supplementation. Parsnips contain a good percentage of folate.

As previously mentioned, parsnips can provide good eye health just like carrots, but how? Parsnips are packed with vitamin C and vitamin E, beta-carotene, and other vitamins that improve eye health and help prevent the development of macular degeneration as we age. You can get parsnips at your local grocery store in the vegetable section, but don't wash them until you are ready to eat them because they lose moisture quickly.

PERSIMMON

Persimmon is an overlooked fruit, similar in appearance to oranges and clementines, and they're sometimes mistaken for tomatoes, but they're very different in taste and flavor. Persimmons are full of antioxidants that fight off free radical damage and help prevent common diseases such as heart disease and diabetes. There are two types of persimmons: one that is an astringent and one that is not. The non-astringent persimmon is very sweet and can be eaten before it is fully ripe; however, the astringent persimmon has a bitter taste before it is ripe and is crunchier.

One of the most important health benefits of persimmon is the high amount of vitamin A it contains. Vitamin A is crucial for eye health and may help prevent blindness, dry eyes, or floaters in the eye. Persimmons contain more than fifty percent of the daily allowance recommended for vitamin A. Persimmons are also packed with fiber, especially the non-astringent ones, aiding in healthy digestion and decreasing the frequency of constipation. They help move unwanted waste out of your digestive system and help increase weight loss.

Lastly, persimmons contain tannins, which are "a class of astringent, polyphenolic biomolecules that bind to and precipitate proteins and various other organic compounds, including amino acids and alkaloids."[180]

Tannins have been known to help prevent high cholesterol, lower blood pressure, and even fight against excessive inflammation in the body, making persimmon, particularly the non-astringent one, a perfect fruit option. You can eat the entire persimmon, including the skin, and it can be used in desserts, main dishes, and as a snack.

DAUGHTER KNOWS BEST

Growing up, I hated zucchini because it was mushy and slimy. But with a mother like mine, whatever she said went, and I had to eat it whether I liked it or not. For years, I hated it and only continued to eat it because I lived in my parents' home. When I grew up, I never bought zucchini. However, my mother called me recently and said she needed to lose weight and had to cut out pasta and bread. The first thing I told her was to buy zucchini. She asked, "Why? What is that going to do?" I told her she could make pasta with zucchini and even use it to make lasagna and substitute it for spaghetti noodles. I have grown to love zucchini, and I eat it weekly. My mother added it as a staple in her diet and lost fifteen pounds after making the switch. Now, she thanks *me* for forcing *her* to eat zucchini; how quickly the tables turn!

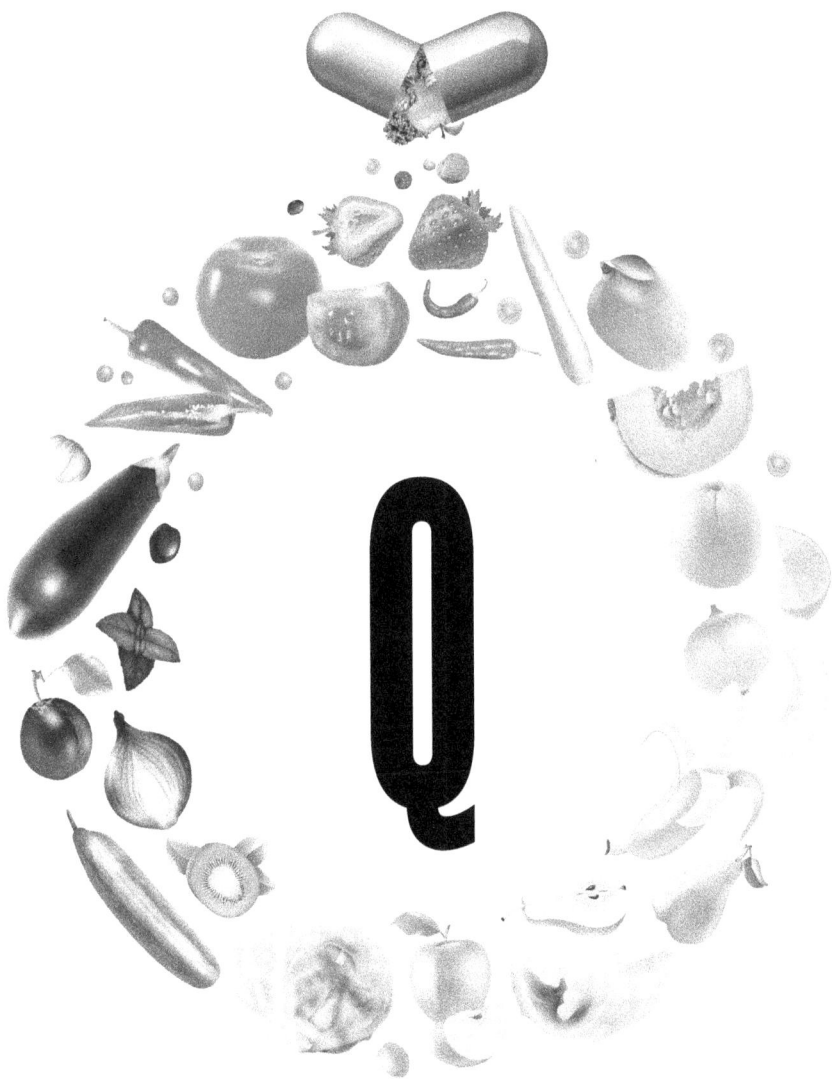

QUINOA

One of the hardest foods for some people to pronounce, Quinoa (Keen-wa) is a seed that is often mistakenly regarded as a grain. It's packed with protein and also happens to be gluten free for my celiac folks. Native to South America, quinoa is so vital because it is one of few plant foods that is a complete protein, meaning it provides us with the twenty essential amino acids we need and even the ones our bodies can't produce on their own. Quinoa has several different varieties and colors, but I appreciate the black quinoa because of the sweeter taste, even though it takes a long time to cook. Let's examine what quinoa can do for us nutritionally and why it should be a staple seed in our pantries.

I mentioned that quinoa is full of essential amino acids. The manganese and magnesium minerals quinoa contains help maintain strong bones and may prevent diabetes and elevated blood sugar levels. Furthermore, manganese may aid in weight loss because it helps the body digest and use food as energy due to the pressure it puts on enzymes and hormones in the body. Quinoa is perfect for helping us shed those few extra pounds we all gain from time to time. Quinoa is fiber rich, giving the feeling of being fuller longer, causing less consumption of food. Also, when we eat more fiber, it allows unwanted toxins to move out of our bodies through the digestive system; therefore, we aren't weighed down and have more energy to move.

What about people who have celiac disease? Quinoa does not contain gluten; therefore, it is a great alternative to rice or other carbohydrates we typically choose to eat. Ever wonder why when you rinse your quinoa, it makes a foam? That's because it contains saponins, which are plant steroids that foam when mixed with water and boast various health benefits. They exhibit anti-inflammatory and immune-boosting properties as well as antibacterial effects. Furthermore, quinoa may help fight cancer and kill cancer cells while maintaining healthy cells.

Cancer contains lunasin, which is an amino acid peptide that binds to the cancer cells chromatin then breaks it.

Quinoa is also full of antioxidants, particularly, quercetin, which fights against chronic inflammation, one of the main causes of diseases we see today, and helps fight free radical damage.[181]

Do you have digestive issues or suffer from Crohn's disease, maybe even irritable bowel syndrome? Quinoa has butyrate,[182] which is a fatty acid our bodies make, but we can also get it from food; it aids in balancing your gut bacteria. It has anti-inflammatory properties that help ward off unwanted toxins and enzymes in the body and fight against colon cancer. Furthermore, butyrate helps regulate the development and production of T-cells in the digestive system. Ultimately, it helps improve the health of the intestines and overall body function. On the other hand, butyrate is also good for the heart. It can slow the production of atherosclerosis or hardening of the arteries in the heart. Quinoa is full of healthy fats, which are good for the heart, and the potassium it has naturally helps lower blood pressure, assisting in better heart health. You can choose red, black or the more common white quinoa to complement your next meal and, ultimately, your body.

Quince

No not a quinceañera—quince, a fruit that's a blend between an apple and a pear. It's native to Hungary, Turkey, and Macedonia and packed with essential vitamins and nutrients in the skin. Quince is filled with antioxidants and phenol compounds that can fight free radical damage and may help prevent cancer by protecting the healthy cells and fighting against non-healthy cell mutation. Quince contains potassium, vitamin A, and calcium, which all help beautify the skin and reduce the presence of wrinkles while fighting off UV radiation damage. When eating fruits and vegetables, you increase your dietary fiber; this aids in weight loss because it helps you feel fuller longer and prevents overeating. Also, fiber helps rid the body of unwanted bacteria and pathogens and keeps the digestive system moving smoothly, decreasing the chances of developing digestive diseases such as irritable bowel disease (IBD) or diverticulitis. On the other hand, its potassium is essential for the body's blood vessels and blood pressure. Potassium helps calm and relax the blood vessels and, in turn, helps decrease the body's blood pressure.

Quince's essential trace elements like iron and zinc are great for the heart because they're necessary for the production of blood cells, and the more red the blood cells, the better circulation throughout the body. Lastly, quince contains vitamin C, which fights inflammation and is great for boosting our immune system naturally to fight bacteria and illnesses and prevent future occurrences. Quince is tart in flavor, so mix it with something sweet if you don't like bitter foods.

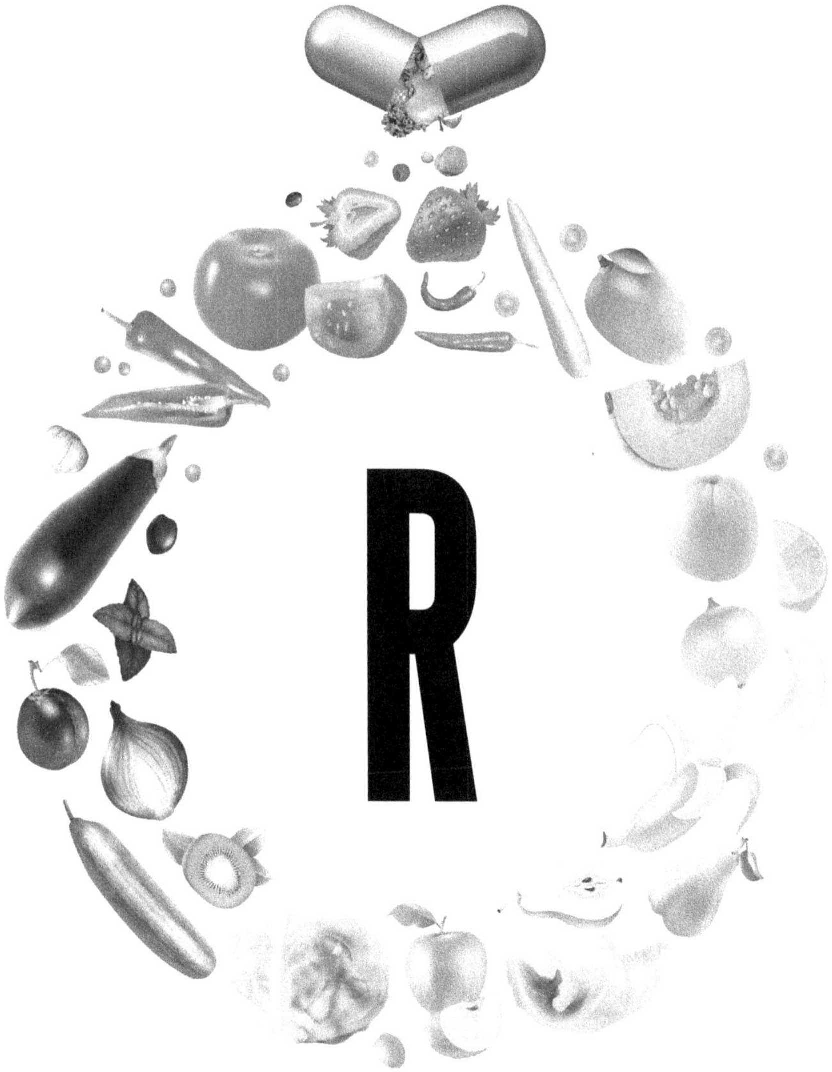
R

RASPBERRIES

Raspberries are delicious when eaten by the handful, in your smoothie, or atop your favorite dessert. Like most berries, raspberries are low in sugar and great for people with type 2 diabetes because they are low on the glycemic index and may help stabilize blood sugar levels. Raspberries contain phytochemicals and antioxidants that not only give them their pigment but also aid in ideal heart health. Let's see what other benefits we receive from raspberries.

With low sugar and the ability to help stabilize sugar levels, raspberries may help you lose weight and increase your metabolism. According to an article from worldhealthfoods.com, "Scientists now know that metabolism in our fat cells can be increased by phytonutrients found in raspberries, especially rheosmin (also called raspberry ketone). By increasing enzyme activity, oxygen consumption, and heat production in certain types of fat cells, raspberry phytonutrients like rheosmin may be able to decrease the risk of obesity as well as the risk of fatty liver. In addition to these benefits, rheosmin can decrease the activity of a fat-digesting enzyme released by our pancreas called pancreatic lipase. This decrease in enzyme activity may result in less digestion and absorption of fat."[183]

Raspberries not only satisfy sugar cravings, but they're also packed with fiber, which helps us eat less throughout the day because we feel fuller longer, and they are slowly digested in the bloodstream.

Do you suffer from arthritis, or are you elderly and want to have great skin? Raspberries have anti-inflammatory properties to help reduce inflammation and pain around the joints. The antioxidants and vitamin C they contain not only fight free radical and sun damage, but they will help improve collagen in the skin and aid in maintaining healthy cells, leaving you with firm, glowing skin.

Remember, when you eat foods with the skin, try to buy organic, and raspberries like the cold, so try to keep them in the fridge so they'll last a little longer.

RAMBUTAN

Many people have never heard of or seen a rambutan. It is similar to lychee fruit and has a spiny exterior but a pale interior with a seed in the middle. Rambutan is full of vitamin C, manganese, fiber, and even contains folate. It's native to Indonesia but can be found in other countries. It has anti-microbial compounds that fight against infections, germs, and viruses while strengthening your immune system to combat them in the future.

Ever experience hemorrhoids, diverticulitis, or an ulcer? These ailments are usually due to a lack of fiber in your diet and poor bowel movements. Fiber helps bulk up the stool, causing a faster rate of movement through the intestines and a decreased chance of unwanted toxins in the body, helping you avoid pain or constipation. Rambutan is also beneficial because it contains several antioxidant properties that help fight against oxidative stress and damage to the body and combat high sugar levels and weight gain; when digested, it slowly absorbs and balances blood sugar.

If you are elderly, have a family history of osteoporosis, or you're at risk for osteopenia, rambutan is your friend. So when you're in the grocery store or farmers market, look for the small red fruit covered in spikes in the exotic or tropical fruit section.

ROSE HIPS

What in the world are we talking about? Rose hips are considered the "false fruit" of the rose plant. You usually see rose hips in fake flower baskets people have in their homes. But rose hips are, indeed, edible and contain a good amount of vitamin C and vitamin A. Vitamin C helps boost our immune system and combat illness and disease while reducing inflammation in the body. Chronic inflammation can affect the body negatively in several was, one being arthritis. Rose hips help relieve pain from arthritis by interfering with the ability of the inflammatory cytokines to activate catabolic proteins like joint tissue degradation.[184]

Rose hips are also good for the skin and help prevent wrinkles with its vitamin C because it helps activate collagen production in the body and maintain healthy cells. If you are diabetic or have a blood disorder or issue, please refrain from supplementing with rose hips.

RADISH

They're red on the outside and have a white, fleshy inside, and they're crunchy like apples but small like cherries. Radishes aren't typically the first vegetable to come to mind when thinking of healthy fruits and vegetables, but did you know radishes help balance your pH levels? Radishes are full of fiber, vitamins A, C, and even B6, which are great nutrients for our bodies that combat constipation, common colds, and illness. They regulate blood pressure and even improve the skin. Let's examine exactly how this works.

Vitamin C aids in fighting against free radical damage, and it's an antioxidant that helps the body produce collagen to improve our skin and reduce inflammation along the joints. Suffer from dry skin or rosacea? Radishes are full of water, aiding in hydration to help remove toxins and impurities from skin. They also contain antibacterial properties that fight against infections in the skin and body.[185]

Do you sometimes get ulcers or infections in the stomach or liver? Radishes contain protein enzymes that help remove any excess bilirubin from your bloodstream while regulating the flow and production of bile, acids, and other enzymes. Want to drop those last few pounds before a big event or party? Radishes are packed with fiber, aiding in proper digestion and removal of waste, leaving no pain or risk of constipation. Furthermore, vegetables with fiber help you reach the feeling of hunger satisfaction sooner, causing a decrease in appetite and consumption of less food throughout the day, aiding in weight loss.

Radishes contain about seven percent of the daily recommended allowance of potassium in one cup, which is ideal for helping to keep blood pressure in check. Radishes help regulate blood pressure by assisting the body in potassium-sodium balance.[186]

You can purchase different types of radishes year round and add them to your favorite salad or side dish.

ROSEMARY

It's one of the best herbs to use on chicken and potatoes, and it has a distinct aroma when passing it outside. Rosemary not only helps make our food taste good, but it helps heal us internally as well. Native to the Mediterranean region, this powerful plant contains antioxidant properties and has purifying effects. Do you have alopecia or severe hair loss? When used in the oil form, it improves hair loss and helps regrow hair. According to a study conducted by Europe PMC, individuals who used rosemary oil on the scalp for approximately six months saw a significant increase in hair count at the six-month endpoint and less scalp itching, providing evidence that rosemary oil is effective in the treatment of alopecia.[187]

Rosemary is great at fighting free radical damage because it contains carnosic acid,[188] which is an ingredient that not only has antioxidant and antimicrobial properties, but also helps protect the brain against damage and improve recovery. Also, a study from the National Institute of Health observed that "Carnosic acid was found to protect fatty acids and triglycerides against oxidation and also was observed to prevent low-density lipoprotein oxidation in human aortic endothelial cells and lipid hydro-peroxide-mediated oxidative stress in other cells,"[189] meaning rosemary helps protect the heart against damage caused from inflammation and stress from outside factors and may help improve cholesterol.

Are you at risk for liver damage, or do you have cirrhosis of the liver? Rosemary has been used for many generations for its healing and medicinal power. It not only aids in cleaning the liver, but also to help heal or improve the functionality. Rosemary is considered a hepato-protective or an herb that helps prevent damage to the liver. Furthermore, it has choleretic[190] effects, which means it can increase the volume of secretion of bile from the liver as well as the amount of solids secreted.

Ever went into a room and thought to yourself, *Why did I come in here?* That's known as a mental fog. I have experienced it before. Rosemary oil can help improve your memory skills and cognitive ability, making you more alert to properly accomplish tasks. A trial study conducted on rosemary oil from the National Institute of Health showed, "Rosemary produced a significant enhancement of performance for overall quality of memory and secondary memory factors but also produced an impairment of speed of memory compared to controls."[191]

If you experience pain, swelling, or inflammation, apply rosemary oil for relief. Whether you choose to cook with rosemary for your favorite foods or you purchase it in the essential oil form, it will provide you significant health benefits.

RHUBARB

Sometimes made into a cake or pie, rhubarb is often mistaken as a fruit, but it is a vegetable. It's packed with antioxidants, which give it its vibrant color and contains many nutrients and vitamins essential for daily life. One essential vitamin Rhubarb contains is vitamin K. We learned earlier that vitamin K is necessary for bone formation, metabolism, density, and health. If you have a family history of weak bones, have been diagnosed with osteoporosis, or you're at risk for osteopenia, rhubarb can help.

Rhubarb contains antioxidants, especially quercetin,[192] a plant pigment or flavonoid that gives vegetables their color. It helps fight against oxidative stress and free radical damage. Antioxidants also help reduce inflammation in the body and organ tissues and protect against unwanted bacteria.

Like most vegetables, rhubarb contains a high amount of fiber. As humans, eighty percent of us do not get in enough daily fiber, which ultimately leads to upset stomach, constipation, and even more serious diagnoses like diverticulitis or colon issues. The high fiber content in rhubarb can assist in getting rid of toxins and waste fast, easing digestion while protecting the intestinal lining and walls. Remember, the leaves of the rhubarb plant are poisonous, but the stalks and flower are great for eating and it tastes best during spring season.

RESVERATROL

You have probably heard that drinking red wine is beneficial for you, but how? Red wine contains resveratrol, which is a powerful bioflavonoid or antioxidant that helps the body combat health problems, and it contains essential phytonutrients. Resveratrol is in wine, but if you are not a wine drinker, it is also in several plants, fruits, and even dark chocolate. It has anti-microbial, antioxidant, and anti-cancer properties to aid in fighting inflammation and free radical damage.

Resveratrol may combat cancer, and based on a study conducted in 2005, "resveratrol blocks the multistep process of carcinogenesis at various stages: tumor initiation, promotion, and progression. One of the possible mechanisms for its biological activities involves down regulation of the inflammatory response through inhibition of synthesis and release of pro-inflammatory mediators, modification of eicosanoid synthesis, and inhibition of activated immune cells."[193]

Resveratrol is good for the heart and can improve circulation while protecting against the formation of atherosclerosis or plaque buildup. Our brain is one of the most important organs in the body, and it's important that we keep it healthy, stimulated, and protected against damage.[194] Resveratrol may increase blood flow to the brain for healthy cognitive function, and it protects the brain because the antioxidants it possesses are able to bypass the blood-brain barrier.

Lastly, resveratrol is considered a phytoestrogen[195] and is beneficial, especially for women who want to get the hormones back in balance during the early stages of menopause. From red wine, to grapes, dark chocolate, and even pistachios, resveratrol is in several of your favorite indulgences and can be a huge benefit to you.

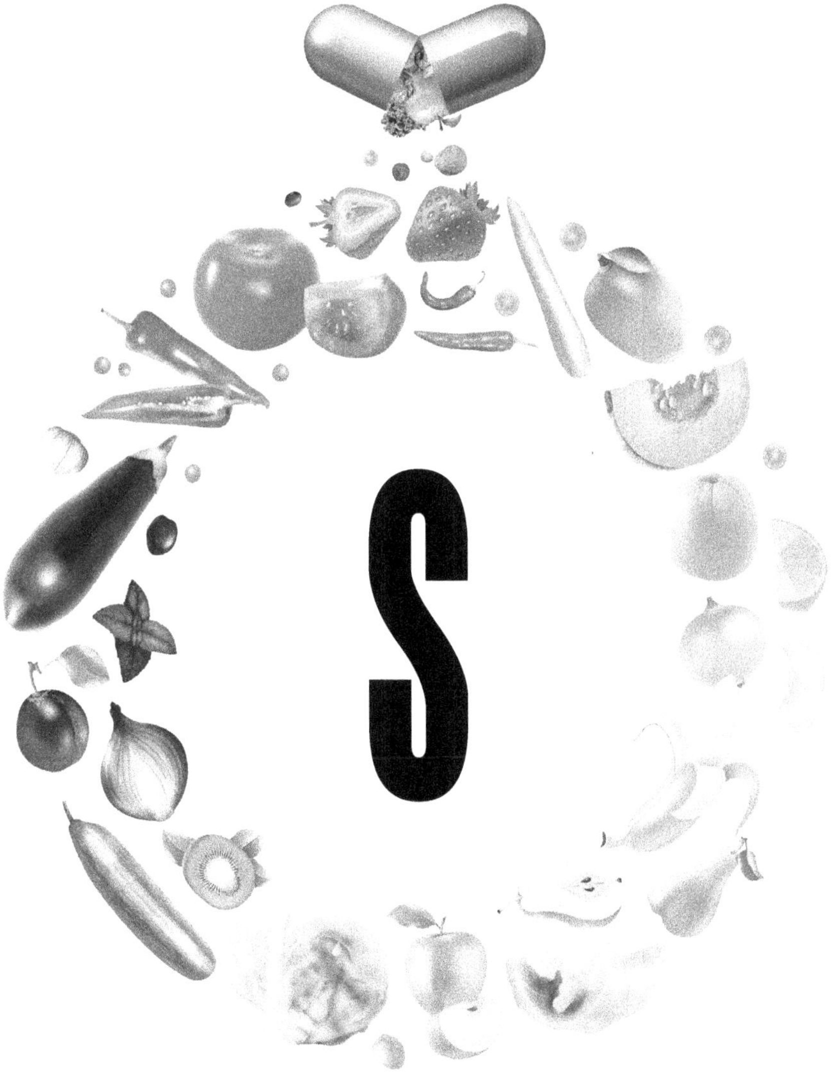

S

SPIRULINA

Often overlooked and even sometimes mistaken for its cousin, chlorella, spirulina is an algae that many people are calling the most nutrient-dense plant in the world. Grown in regions from Hawaii to Africa, spirulina is a necessary plant to include in your daily dietary regimen. From boosting energy to helping to balance blood sugar levels, improving digestion and lowering cholesterol levels, this plant can profoundly improve your overall body function. Maintaining a good internal microbial health is essential to our metabolic health. *How so?* Microbes and fungi are one of the leading reasons individuals face illness and disease. Diseases such as IBS, leaky gut, yeast infections, and many others are due to a buildup of unhealthy bacteria in the body. For us women, it is important to maintain good vaginal health and gut health, especially since we bear children. Luckily, spirulina is an antimicrobial that helps inhibit bacteria such as candida and help promote good gut flora and microbial health while boosting your immune system.[196]

Do you have high cholesterol, so you've been trying to eat healthy and exercise regularly but your numbers are stagnant? Try adding spirulina into your diet; it has hypocholesterolemic properties and the ability to assist your body in fighting off other heart-related diseases.[197] One study was conducted to determine spirulina effects on mice that had high cholesterol compared to a group that were not fed spirulina, and the results shocked me. The results suggested that spirulina intake can cause the reduction of hypercholesterolemic atherosclerosis associated with a decrease in levels of serum TC, TG, and LDL-C and an elevation of HDL-C level.[198] Spirulina may, therefore, be beneficial in preventing atherosclerosis and reducing risk factors for cardiovascular diseases.

Do you have clean water? Is your water filtered, and if so, are the pollutants and contaminants really removed? Arsenic poisoning is a big issue in several countries that don't have access to clean water. Spirulina, however, has been tested on its ability to help remove toxins and heavy metals like arsenic from the body. One study conducted in Bangladesh was performed on people who had been affected by arsenic poisoning and tested how taking spirulina with zinc would hurt or help their conditions. The results indicated that spirulina extract plus zinc removed 47.1 percent arsenic from scalp hair, and using it twice daily for sixteen weeks may be useful for the treatment of chronic arsenic poisoning with melanosis and keratosis.[199]

Spirulina also exhibits anti-inflammatory properties by inhibiting the release of histamine from mast cells. Chronic inflammation in the body can cause serious problems and damage, often leading to disease; however, consuming spirulina may combat inflammation and fight free radical damage.[200]

Whether you choose to mix it with water, add it to your favorite smoothie, or cook with it, supplementing with plant-based products like spirulina is the best way to maintain great health.

SEAWEED

The typical green stuff you find in sushi, its grown in the ocean, and it's sometimes even eaten raw as a snack or chips. Seaweed is a versatile, nutritious food. Specifically, wakame seaweed is full of minerals such as potassium, iodine, and iron. Foods containing iron help improve blood production and fight against iron deficiency.[201] Also, iodine is essential for the thyroid, which controls hormones, balances reproduction, and helps repair cells.[202] Just one sheet of wakame seaweed contains almost ninety-five percent of the recommended daily allowance of iodine. Looks like I am going to eat more seaweed.

Family history of osteoporosis? Seaweed contains calcium. Calcium not only helps strengthen our bones, but it increases the rate of repair when damage is present. When pregnant, folate and B12 are the most essential nutrients needed for a healthy baby. Folate helps prevent issues like spina bifida and neural defects. Wakame seaweed contains folate, which is necessary for DNA replication and proper immune function, even creating new cells, not just for expecting moms but everyone.

Wakame seaweed, native to the Asian culture, is packed with antioxidants and carotenoids. One prominent carotenoid present is fucoxanthin. This carotenoid may be better for cell production than vitamin A. Your body absorbs it best when eaten with some form of fat. No wonder sushi is usually made with this seaweed and spicy mayo!

One study conducted on mice showed wakame seaweed may not only help combat diabetes but may also help prevent obesity. The mice's adipose tissue (fat) improved, and their blood sugar improved when incorporating wakame seaweed into their diets.[203]

On the other hand, seaweed contains several antioxidants that fight against free radical damage and help improve and maintain healthy cells.

Ever had sushi or seaweed chips and a few hours later, you had to use the restroom? Seaweed is full of fiber, and most of its weight is fiber! Fiber is necessary for good gut health and aids in proper digestion. It helps remove unwanted toxins and provides ease when releasing stool. Fiber also helps you feel fuller longer, meaning you may lose weight due to a decrease of appetite and cravings.

Seaweed's carotenoid fucoxanthin also activates the liver to produce DHA, therefore aiding in the reduction of "bad cholesterol" and unwanted plaque in the body.[204]

Remember, seaweed is best absorbed with a fat, and you can eat it raw or cooked and receive great health benefits.

STRAWBERRIES

Nice, big, red, and juicy, strawberries are one of the most loved fruits, and they're versatile; they're used in breakfast and snacks, even desserts. But strawberries are not really berries. *Say what?* I will explain later. Just know they are an aggregate fruit.

First, we'll break down the health benefits, from inflammation to weight loss and help with diabetes and cholesterol. *Why are strawberries perfect for summer and so refreshing?* Well, during the summer, we are outside more often. The sun causes damage to our skin, dehydrates us, and accelerates the aging process. Strawberries contain several antioxidants that fight against free radical damage and oxidative stress on the body that we face from the sun and environmental factors that are out of our control. Also, strawberries contain vitamin C, which is great for building the immune system and aiding collagen production to give us glowing skin and reduce hyperpigmentation and wrinkles.

Strawberries contain the antioxidant anthocyanin and may fight against cancer cell production and replication and may inhibit the progression of the cells while leaving healthy cells intact. Trying to lose weight or just get more fruit into your diet? Strawberries are considered one of the lower-sugar fruits, and they contain fiber, so not only are they a good option when dieting, but they will keep you full as well. Fiber helps detoxify the body, promote regularity, decrease chronic inflammation, and aids in proper gut health, so strawberries are ideal for fighting against constipation or even ulcers.

Do you have high cholesterol or are you at risk for heart disease? Strawberries are low in sugar and a great fruit option because they may stop the oxidation of LDL or the "bad cholesterol" in the body. Furthermore, they aid in proper blood flow and reduce plaque buildup in the arterial wall and arteries. Strawberries contain folate and manganese, which is ideal for pregnant women to help decrease birth defects, and we need it to help with DNA replication, proper cell function, and rebuilding tissues. *Well, what about manganese?* We need this trace mineral for bone health and proper brain health and cognition. Manganese is great for making our veins bigger so they can carry blood to the brain and other vital organs. It may help reduce the presence of seizures since one of the main causes of seizures may be due to a decrease in manganese.

I mentioned that strawberries aren't a fruit, and you were probably puzzled. Fun fact: Strawberries come from a flower that contains ovaries, and every seed is an ovary with a seed inside of it. Crazy, I know. So whether you eat strawberries because you like the taste or for health reasons, enjoy them in abundance!

SPINACH

Kale has recently replaced spinach in popularity, but it is a nutrient-dense vegetable. It contains very few calories, but it's packed with flavonoids, phytonutrients, and vitamins that can help fight against disease and aging and reduce inflammation in the body. Full of antioxidants, spinach may help fight cellular damage and provide energy to combat illness. The number one vitamin in spinach is vitamin K, which is necessary for proper bone development and maintaining good bone health. Vitamin K helps reduce the risk of developing osteopenia or osteoporosis and helps combat degradation of the brain and cognitive function typically caused by inflammation.

Do you suffer from pain or cramps frequently? Are you taking a multivitamin that contains magnesium? Magnesium deficiency affects thousands of people around the world, and some don't even know they're deficient. Spinach is full of magnesium, which is necessary for the stimulation of calcium uptake in the body and has a part in body functions and muscular contractions. One article stated, "Magnesium critically stabilizes enzymes, including many ATP-generating reactions. ATP is required universally for glucose utilization, synthesis of fat, proteins, nucleic acids and coenzymes, muscle contraction, methyl group transfer and many other processes, and interference with magnesium metabolism also influences these functions. Thus, one should keep in mind that ATP metabolism, muscle contraction and relaxation, normal neurological function and release of neurotransmitters are all magnesium dependent. It is also important to note that magnesium contributes to the regulation of vascular tone, heart rhythm, platelet-activated thrombosis and bone formation."[205]

One of the main causes of several diseases is chronic inflammation and oxidative stress on the body and body systems. The antioxidants and carotenoids present in spinach help fight against disease and maybe even cancer because they block oxidative stress and DNA damage.

It is important for us to take care of our heart. The heart is a muscle, and it must be exercised and have proper blood flow. Spinach's flavonoids help protect against cardiovascular damage and disease. The flavonoids augment nitric oxide, which helps to improve heart tissue, lower blood pressure, and improve function. From high cholesterol to high blood pressure and atherosclerosis, the antioxidants and nutrients in spinach help keep healthy blood flow, combat plaque buildup on the arterial lining and walls, and lower inflammation and blood pressure.

High blood sugar? Yeah, let's talk about it. Many Americans are battling diabetes or just trying to stabilize their blood sugar and lose weight. One of the key factors in weight loss is maintaining good sugar levels and preventing constant drops and spikes. Spinach contains a steroid—the good kind—called phytoecdysteroid. It helps with stabilizing blood sugar and metabolizing glucose.[206] This is very important for diabetic patients who are already at risk for developing complications such as blindness, loss of limbs, and even heart damage.[207]

Also, spinach is full of fiber, which can help reduce fasting glucose and, in turn, lower A1C levels. Foods high in fiber are also great for digestive health, as they aid in removing unwanted toxins and pathogens in the body.[208]

Diverticulosis, chronic constipation, and ulcers can occur due to a lack of adequate fiber and good gut bacteria in the body. Spinach has phytonutrients that can help cleanse the gut and maintain good gut flora while removing unnecessary bacteria and reducing inflammation.[209]

Looking for a quick fix for a cold or are you always getting sick? Spinach contains vitamins A and C, which will help boost your immunity to combat illness. These vitamins fight against bacteria and replicate what caused you to become sick to help prevent it from occurring again. Furthermore, vitamin A is great for eye health, improving the retina and reducing the risk of eye diseases such as macular degeneration.[210]

Spinach also contains carotenoids that are essential for the eye. "Lutein and zeaxanthin have been shown to filter high-energy wavelengths of visible light and act as antioxidants to protect against the formation of reactive oxygen species and subsequent free radicals."[211] These carotenoids protect against UV light, oxidative stress, and any other complications known to the eye.[212]

Want that glowing, radiant skin? With its vitamin C, spinach helps foster the production of collagen and the growth of new skin cells, aiding in youthful looking skin.[213]

I love my spinach in a smoothie or a salad; however, some like it cooked. Whichever method you prefer, enjoy the benefits it offers.

SESAME SEEDS

Atop your favorite salad, drizzled on your sushi roll, and even roasted for a boost of flavor for that amazing main dish, sesame seeds are versatile, high-flavor seeds that provide healthy fat and are packed with nutrients. Sesame seeds may help lower blood pressure. A study from the *Yale Journal of Biology & Medicine* was conducted on the effects sesame seeds and oil had on patients with high blood pressure. "In the present study, substitution of sesame oil lowered systolic and diastolic blood pressure remarkably in hypertensive patients. Studies reported that sesamin, a lignan from sesame oil, exerts antihypertensive action by interfering with renin-angiotensin system."[214]

Sesame seeds contain several vital benefits. They have lots of iron and fiber, which helps with iron deficiency and may prevent constipation and improve gut health. Furthermore, its manganese, protein, and polyphenols may help lower cholesterol and improve heart function and energy while helping to balance levels, and the fiber helps prevent the frequency of spikes and drops in the blood sugar.

Sesame seeds, we know, contain fat, but it's the good fat we need to absorb fat soluble vitamins like vitamins D, K, and E. Sesame seeds are ideal for women because they may balance sex hormones, and as women, those hormones fluctuate like crazy. A study was conducted on postmenopausal women to see how sesame seeds could improve their overall health. The results indicated that sesame benefits postmenopausal women by improving blood lipids, antioxidant status, and possibly sex hormone status.[215]

Has someone you know passed away from cancer? Just about everyone knows a family member or friend who has succumbed to the horrible disease. Sesame seeds may have an effect on cancer cells in the body. A study was performed on women with breast cancer and women without breast cancer, and the results showed that higher lignan intake was associated with lower risks of breast cancer. The study also showed that lignans may affect breast cancer by modifying tumor characteristics likely to affect prognosis.[216] Sesame seeds cannot cure cancer, and each person's body responds differently to foods and treatment, but the lignans sesame seeds contain may help decrease your chances of developing the disease.[217]

Just remember, eating sesame seeds raw is best; cooking them breaks down several of the seeds' nutrients.

SAFFLOWER OIL

Typically, we know oil is needed in the diet but in moderation, and only certain types of oil are good for you. There are two types of safflower oil; one is considered a high-oleic, which is ideal for cooking at high smoke points, e.g., stir-fry. The other type is high-linoleic, which is perfect for a salad dressing and not used for cooking. Safflower oil comes from the safflower plant and is considered an unsaturated fat, meaning this oil is great for you, allowing your body to absorb fat-soluble vitamins, and it helps the regulation of hormones and brain function. Furthermore, safflower oil is great for the heart, helping to reduce plaque buildup and improve cholesterol, and it reduces chronic inflammation throughout the body. It helps grease the lining of the arterial walls, and platelets, in turn, are less clammy or stuck together to help prevent unnecessary clotting, decreasing your chances of heart disease or a stroke.[218]

Do you moisturize your body with oil or lotion? I used to use lotion and body cream, but I am strictly an oil woman now. Safflower oil helps moisturize the skin, protects cells from environmental and sun damage, and combats free radical damage with the vitamin E it contains. Vitamin E helps decrease the appearance of scars and soothe dry skin, which is great for people who suffer from eczema, and it may even help improve psoriasis.[219]

Safflower oil is a good oil option for those who want to lose weight without cutting the oil. Safflower oil is *not* a low-calorie food; however, adding a small portion of the oil helps bring out bold flavors from the food you're cooking, so you may eat less and feel more satisfied quicker. In all aspects of use for safflower oil, test with a small amount and see how your body responds.

SAFFRON

The most expensive spice in the world, saffron is native to Europe, and a little goes a long way. It not only adds flavor to your food, but it also adds benefits to your body. Let's examine some of the benefits. Saffron contains the carotenoid crocin,[220] and it has been known to have an aphrodisiac effect on humans.

Many men have difficulty achieving erections, but saffron may help with erectile dysfunction. A study was performed on men with ED, and after ten days of taking a few hundred milligrams of saffron, the men had an increase in swelling or turgid improvement of the tip and an increase in the rigidity of the base.[221]

Hundreds of thousands of people deal with mental illness, and it is becoming a more frequently discussed topic along with ways to help individuals cope. Saffron may help with depression and have a more positive effect than pharmaceutical medication. In a study conducted with individuals who have major depression disorder, saffron was used as a relief option versus antidepressants. The results of the study showed that saffron supplementation significantly reduced depression symptoms compared to the placebo control.[222]

Also, saffron may help with cramps and PMS because it can regulate or control muscle spasms.[223] I have experienced bad cramps before and during my cycle, so when I learned saffron could help, I was ecstatic.

Lastly, saffron is packed with several compounds that act as antioxidants, helping to fight against oxidative stress and free radical damage. Furthermore, these compounds aid in chronic inflammation and protect against cell damage. Even though it is an expensive spice, try to buy it as often as needed to help you and your food.

SAGE

As an herb, it is commonly used in small amounts but packed with big nutrients. Sage contains several polyphenols or plant compounds that act as antioxidants in the body. Antioxidants help combat cellular damage, chronic inflammation, and oxidative stress from free radical damage. High cholesterol is a common diagnosis for many Americans today, and we are always looking for ways to lower those numbers. Sage may decrease the LDL or "bad" cholesterol while improving the HDL or "good" cholesterol. A study was conducted on healthy individuals to see what effects sage as a tea would have on them. The results indicated an improvement in lipid profile, lower plasma LDL cholesterol and total cholesterol levels, as well as higher plasma HDL cholesterol levels during and after treatment. Drinking sage tea regularly may be the key to improving those cholesterol numbers.[224]

Sage contains antimicrobial properties and may fight against fungus and microbes. One of the biggest places we hold microbes is in our mouths, and drinking sage tea or even using a mouthwash with sage in it can combat those germs.[225]

The compounds in sage may improve our memory, cognitive function, and overall brain health. As we age, some of us develop dementia or Alzheimer's disease, which is characterized as a decrease in cognitive function. Sage compounds may stop the breakdown of (ACH) or Acetylcholine, which is usually low in individuals with Alzheimer's. A study was conducted on patients with mild to moderate Alzheimer's who were administered sixty drops of sage per day for four months to measure the effects on their cognition. The treatment produced a significantly better outcome on cognitive functions than the placebo.[226]

Sage contains about ten percent of the recommended daily allowance of vitamin K in just one teaspoon and helps maintain strong bones, protect against bone fractures, and increases the rate of bone repair. Many people burn sage as a way to cleanse or remove any negative energy from a space and generate wisdom. Whether you are burning sage, using it as an oil, or adding it to your foods, remember, sage is more than just an herb; it is a powerhouse that helps us internally and externally.

SUNFLOWER LECITHIN

Lecithin? What is it? Lecithin is a substance found naturally in our body tissues. Lecithin also comes in the form of many foods and is even used as an additive to foods and food products. Soy and corn lecithin are the most common forms; however, they're not necessarily the best for you. Sunflower lecithin has several health benefits that we will briefly discuss.

It may improve cognitive function and brain health. It contains choline, which is a nutrient needed for brain health and a precursor for ACH (acetylcholine). Digestive issues are a big concern in the United States and for people worldwide, but sunflower lecithin may help relieve pain associated with Crohn's disease, irritable bowel syndrome, and diverticulitis or diverticulosis. A study conducted in 2013 showed that lecithin accounted for more than seventy percent of total phospholipids within the intestinal mucus layer, and it helps to prevent invasion of the colonic commensal microbiota.[227] Therefore, lecithin may help block and prevent unwanted bacteria and microbes from entering the digestive system.

Many women suffer from excessive pain while breastfeeding, even experiencing breast engorgement. However, lecithin can aid in reducing clogged milk ducts, pain, and inflammation while breastfeeding. Sunflower lecithin also helps with the absorption of fat-soluble vitamins and is packed with nutrients such as calcium, phosphorus, and Iron.[228]

You can purchase sunflower lecithin at your local grocery store or farmers market in the vitamin section.

STEVIA

Is it sugar, or is it artificial sweetener? Actually, stevia is an herbal plant native to Brazil that is naturally sweet. It is a sweetener that can be used instead of artificial sugar, and it's made up of two glycosides: sativoside and rebaudioside.[229] *Is it good to use sweetener instead of real sugar? It's natural, so it is good, right?* We are going to dig a little deeper to answer those questions.

The stevia plant is natural, but make sure you're not buying the processed version. The closest form to the real thing we can purchase in the States is stevia leaf extract; however, in places like Japan, if you find green leaf stevia, it is the best type to purchase. Stevia may fight against cancer, specifically breast cancer. One study showed stevia reduced certain pathways of stress that usually aid in cancer growth and sativoside may augment cancer cell death.[230]

Furthermore, stevia may help in weight loss and even lower blood pressure. Certain compounds found in stevia may open blood vessels and amplify sodium emission, things that are part of keeping good blood pressure.[231]

Sugar is one of the main reasons it is hard to lose weight, but using stevia as a no-calorie sweetener will not spike your blood sugar, and it will help you lose weight while combating sugar cravings. Just remember to read the label before purchasing any stevia or stevia-related products, and make sure it's stevia leaf extract without fillers.

STONE ROOT

With many different names such as collinsonia root, stone root has a few health benefits you may not be aware of. First, stone root is a plant native to North America and was first used for medicinal purposes in the 1800s. This root contains plant flavonoids and saponins that have anti-inflammatory and anti-microbial effects, making it ideal to combat illnesses, boost immune function and improve overall metabolic health.[232]

The most common use of stone root is to help relieve the pain associated with hemorrhoids. Due to its anti-inflammatory effects, stone root can help reduce the swelling and bleeding associated with hemorrhoids while coating the lining of the rectum and anus. It can also help support the uprightness of blood vessels with the saponins it contains, which is ideal for individuals who suffer from varicose veins.[233] From improving heart health and overall blood circulation, stone root is a versatile herb.

Suffer from upper respiratory infections, bronchitis, or laryngitis? Stone root is considered a mucous membrane tonic herb, making it great for improving the function and tone of the throat and esophageal tract while decreasing irritation.[234]

Not commonly used, stone root has several benefits we can utilize frequently. Just remember, stone root has a pungent, unpleasant odor, and it could be called something else when you're looking for it at the store, so make sure you read the label.

S T. JOHN'S WORT

Used for over 2000 years for its medicinal properties, St. John's wort has antidepressant and anti-inflammatory properties. It originated in Europe and is beneficial due to the many plant compounds it contains, so much that it is now widely grown in the U.S. and other countries.[235] One of the main benefits of St. John's wort is its ability to help relieve mild depression and anxiety. Scientists are still researching how it is able to do this, but some have concluded that its due to the effect it has on neurotransmitters in our brain like serotonin that affects our mood. Some even believe St. John's wort has comparable affects to Prozac with the way it helps enhance our mood and relieve depression.[236]

As women age, their hormones and moods can shift at the drop of a dime; therefore, it is important to never say the wrong thing too quickly. However, St. John's wort positively affects our mood, providing relief to others and may improve psychological symptoms in menopausal women. One study noted that women who had menopausal symptoms such as mood changes and fatigue took St. John's wort over a period of twelve weeks and showed substantial improvement in psychological and psychosomatic symptoms.[237]

Also, St. John's wort may help combat cancer. It contains a bio-active compound called hyperforin,[238] which induces apoptosis in tumor cells to inhibit cancer invasion and metastasis. These anti-cancer properties may help diminish or eliminate cancerous cells in the body.

Do you have eczema like me, or do you cut or bruise easily? When applied topically, St. John's wort may help increase the rate of healing and decrease the size of bruises or visible irritation due to its anti-inflammatory properties. According to a study conducted on several patients with atopic dermatitis or eczema, when used as a cream, St. John's wort caused improvement in the intensity of the eczematous lesions and areas of the skin that had bacteria such as staph. St. John's wort's anti-bacterial properties can help with skin lesions and reduce inflammation internally and externally.[239]

Ever wonder where the name St. John's wort came from? I did, and I found out the name is derived from the fact that the flower blooms around the summer solstice or St. Johns Day, June 24. Quite interesting.

SAW PALMETTO

Before I started writing this book, I didn't know what saw palmetto was, but I quickly learned. Saw Palmetto extract comes from the saw palmetto palm tree. It has been used by Native Americans for many years, and now, it is more readily found and used for its medicinal purposes and health benefits.

Men, this is for you, so pay attention because we'll cover topics that may concern you as you age. Saw palmetto may help with hair loss and thinning as you get older.[240] Hair loss is due to the hair follicles' sensitivity to dihydrotestosterone (DHT), which is a male sex androgen hormone. This causes the hair to diminish and fall out. Typically, the hair will re-grow unless the presence of DHT is high.[241]

As men age, the amount of testosterone in the body decreases significantly. *Okay, great. What does this have to do with saw palmetto?* Well, it has the ability to inhibit the conversion of testosterone into DHT. Furthermore, saw palmetto is great for women and men who suffer from weakened bladders or urinary organs, especially women who have had large babies that may have pushed things around. It strengthens the urinary tract receptors. One study suggested that saw palmetto improves urologic symptoms and flow measures comparable to finasteride but with fewer adverse treatment events.[242]

Saw palmetto may assist men who have engorged or enlarged prostates, causing urinary pain to the point of an infection. Saw palmetto may block testosterone from attaching to and stimulating prostate cells, which may lead to improved prostate and urinary function. According to a study conducted on several men who had BPH (benign prostate hypertrophy), saw palmetto as a treatment showed improvement in BPH symptoms.[243]

Lastly, saw palmetto may maintain normal testosterone levels and improve energy; however, every individual is different. You can purchase saw palmetto extract at your local health food store or even at a vitamin store.

SPAGHETTI SQUASH

An option for making your favorite pasta dish or having Italian night at home, spaghetti squash has recently become a staple in many homes. If you are trying to reduce your carbohydrate consumption without losing flavor or missing your favorite meals, spaghetti squash may be the option for you. It is a nutrient-dense vegetable that's low in calories and high in fiber and vitamin C.[244] When cooked, it resembles traditional spaghetti pasta, so your kids may not even recognize that they're eating a vegetable instead of pasta. It's a great mom hack!

Spaghetti squash is full of antioxidants, which are known to fight against free radical damage and oxidative stress while protecting our body and cells. The vitamin C it contains aids in boosting the immune system to better fight off disease and aims to help combat illnesses you face daily. From atherosclerosis to the common cold and even cancer, antioxidants are crucial to help maintain healthy cell function and disease prevention.

Are you looking to lose weight, or do you suffer from diabetes, and you're trying to make healthier food choices? Spaghetti squash contains about forty calories per cup and about six grams of carbohydrates, making it great for dieters. Because its low in sugar, it will not cause a spike in blood sugar levels, and it's great for maintaining balance in overall health numbers for diabetic individuals. The fiber in spaghetti squash adds bulk to your stool, making digestion a breeze and helps prevent digestive issues like constipation, GERD, hemorrhoids, and ulcers.[245]

Fiber helps you feel fuller longer and coats the lining of the intestines, making bowel movements less painful. When cooking spaghetti squash, remember to put a little oil on the flesh part and season to your liking. Turn it open side down and cook until tender. Remove with a fork and enjoy!

STAR FRUIT

Known mostly for its appearance, star fruit is more than just a pretty face. It is a versatile fruit native to Vietnam and the Philippines and may help reduce inflammation, fight against illness, and help you lose weight, just to name a few benefits. Averrhoa carambola L. (Oxalidaceae), an Asian tree that was introduced to Brazil, is also known as the star fruit tree and is commonly used to treat headaches, vomiting, coughing, and hangovers. The extract obtained through decocting the leaves has been used to treat diabetes.

Star fruit contains several antioxidants and complex compounds needed to combat disease and fight free radical damage in the body. Star fruit has quercetin,[246] which is a flavonoid that may reduce inflammation and improve athletic performance by increasing endurance. "The insoluble fibers of the star fruit slow the absorption of carbohydrates, significantly reducing blood glucose levels. The fiber can also act to prevent cardiovascular disease by reducing serum triglyceride and total cholesterol levels."[247]

Star fruit is also great for people who suffer from frequent constipation, have diverticulitis, or are at risk for diverticulosis due to the high fiber content it possesses. Fiber is needed for a proper digestive health, removal of unwanted toxins, and adequate good gut bacteria.

Star fruit contains vitamin C, helping to combat diseases and respiratory infections. Vitamin C boosts our immune system to fight illness and helps our helper T cells replicate a virus to further help us avoid that illness again. Star fruit has more than fifty percent of our daily vitamin C, so it is a great option if you have an allergy to oranges or just want a change in your dietary routine.[248]

Star fruit, low in sugar and calories but high in fiber, is ideal for weight loss, keeping you fuller longer and decreasing the frequency of hunger cravings. Get variety in your diet by adding star fruit for added health benefits.

REAL FOOD, REAL RESULTS

My cousin was always on the heavier side growing up. She loved to eat and didn't see the importance of making healthy choices. As she went into adulthood, her weight continued to increase, and she developed severe self-esteem issues. The only form of exercise she did was dancing on the weekends and a brisk walk to and from her car as she went to work and home. One day, the doctor informed her that she was at risk for developing diabetes if she didn't change her eating habits. She wasn't happy but said she would give it a try. She went from one fad diet to the next, losing weight then gaining it back. Nothing worked. I reached out to her because I saw that she was struggling. I advised her to eat "real" food, to put down the processed and fast food and not to limit or starve herself. I advised her to choose foods that would nourish her body and keep her full. She began eating lean meats, green vegetables, and she even began fasting. In time, she realized she loved fats and was not a fan of heavy carbohydrates, so the keto lifestyle was best for her. She has not only lost 130 pounds, but she has kept it off. She balances her lifestyle with occasional cheat meals and lots of water. She learned that it's not about limiting herself or cutting out food groups, but balancing the food she loves with her new healthy lifestyle.

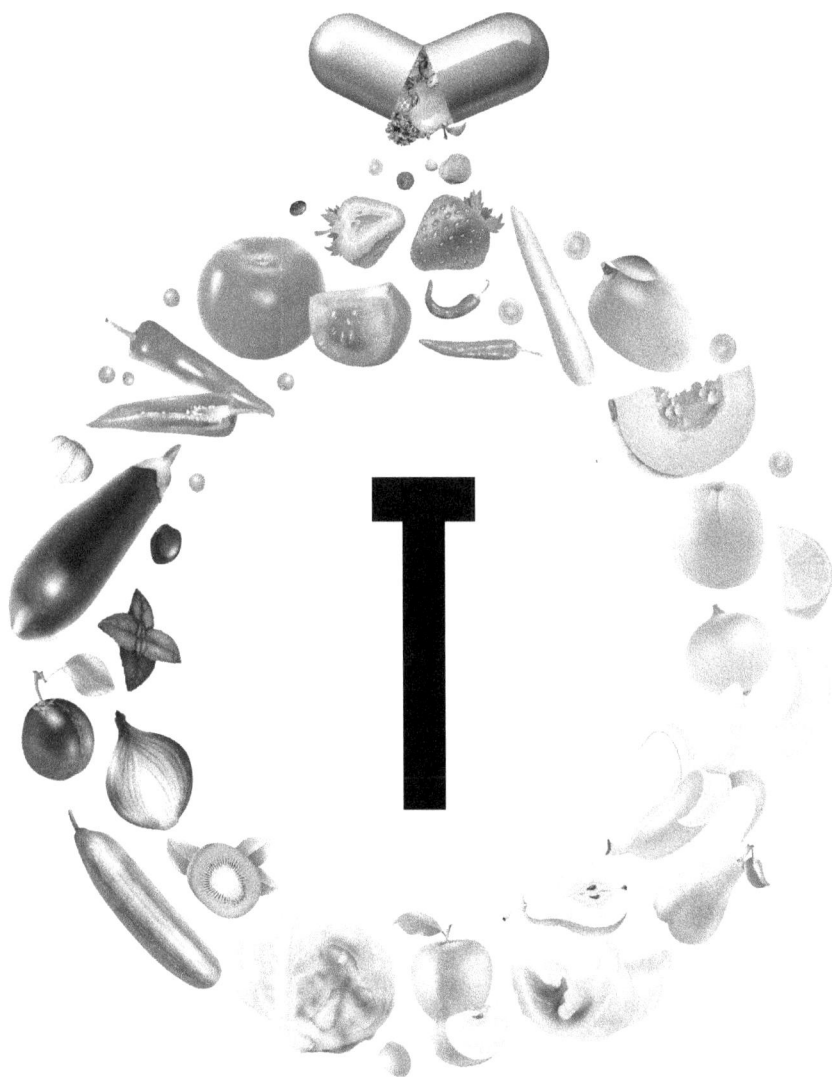

TOMATO

From grape to roma, and even vine ripened, tomatoes are an excellent fruit—yes, fruit. And they provide numerous health benefits. Tomatoes contain a nutrient called lycopene[249] and are full of vitamin K, vitamin C, and folate. As an anti-inflammatory, tomatoes may help fight against certain cancers, aid in bone health, and combat disease and infections. The older we get, the more common it is to experience a decline in bone health and degradation; however, vitamin K is essential to the development of bone health and maintenance. Tomatoes are great for salads and as a snack, but they provide even more benefits when cooked because the heat allows a more intense release of lycopene. A trial conducted on men who ate tomatoes or tomato sauce showed that consumption of two to four servings of tomato sauce per week was associated with a thirty-five percent risk reduction of total prostate cancer and a fifty percent reduction of advanced (extraprostatic) prostate cancer.[250] Therefore, tomatoes may be a great addition to help combat prostate cancer and inhibit the formation of cancerous compounds in the body.

As I mentioned, tomatoes are an anti-inflammatory, and this is especially important for the heart. If you have experienced heart problems or have a family history of heart disease, tomatoes combat free radical damage and oxidative stress, which is one of the main causes of heart disease today. One of the antioxidants tomatoes contains is lutein,[251] and it may help prevent high cholesterol by helping to slow down arterial wall thickening. Also, lutein helps improve eye health and decrease the chance of developing macular degeneration or cataracts, and it protects the eye against UV or sun damage.

Do you hate bananas, and you're worried you aren't getting enough potassium? Tomatoes are a potassium-rich food and provide nearly nine percent of the daily recommended allowance. In addition, its vitamin C not only helps fight illness and disease, but it's also great for maintaining healthy skin. From eczema to hyperpigmentation and even stubborn acne, tomatoes' carotenoid lutein allows you to have glowing skin, improved elasticity, and a decrease in wrinkles.[252]

Whether you use tomatoes to make your family's secret spaghetti, add them to your favorite salad, or use them to top your tostados for taco night, enjoy plenty of tomatoes.

TANGERINES

Packaged as Cuties or sometimes mistaken for oranges, tangerines have a thin exterior, making them easy to peel, and can be sweeter than oranges. Also, they are small in size, ideal for a great snack. They have vital nutrients and vitamins we need daily while curbing sweet cravings.

Tangerines received their name because they are originally from the city of Tangier in Morocco. Tangerines, like oranges, contain vitamin C to help improve and strengthen our immune system and are packed with vitamin A, which is essential for proper eye health. Tangerines are high in fiber and ideal for weight loss or relieving constipation.[253]

The antioxidants they contain combat free radical damage, which typically causes diseases. Just like oranges, tangerines are great for a post-workout snack and help combat high cholesterol or severe inflammation throughout the body. Tangerines are the "mini" oranges, and children love them!

TAMARIND

The first time I heard the word "tamarind," I thought, *What is that?* Tamarind is a fruit that comes from a tree native to Africa. It's also grown in other parts of the world and has a unique pod shape. It can be used in your favorite dish and dessert as a complement. From improving digestion to combating illness and improving the heart, tamarind has an array of benefits.[254]

Tamarind is considered an antioxidant and anti-inflammatory due to the plant phenols it contains, which combat free radical damage and oxidative stress. It helps decrease chronic inflammation and fight against illnesses like bronchitis and arthritis. Also, tamarind has antimicrobial and antibacterial effects due to its lupeol content.[255]

Tamarind is high in fiber and helps ease digestion and relieve constipation. Fiber is necessary to help rid the body of unwanted waste and toxins while promoting weight loss. Foods high in magnesium help maintain healthy bone density, promote good heart health, and help with muscle contractions.[256]

Tamarind contains about twenty-seven percent of the daily recommended allowance for magnesium. Although Tamarind is fairly high in calories, it is a great substitute for a dessert when you're trying to watch your weight.

TARRAGON

Not often considered for cooking or seasoning your favorite dish, tarragon is a great herb to use for added flavor, but it's also great for medicinal purposes. From bloating to tooth decay and even infections, tarragon can help relieve pain and decrease the chances of developing the aforementioned ailments. With food, the digestion process starts when we smell the food and our mouths start salivating before the food even enters the body. The carotenoids in tarragon aids with proper digestion and expedites the gastric juices to digest food more rapidly. Also, when tarragon is transformed into an essential oil, it has antibacterial effects and may combat staph and E. coli. According to the results of a study from the National Institute of Health, tarragon essential oil has antibacterial effects to treat S. aureus and E. coli.[257]

Do you have sleep apnea or struggle staying asleep? Tarragon, when made into a tea, can help calm the body and soothe the organs and organ tissues to help promote better sleep. Tarragon contains the compound eugenol, which is known to help relieve pain and inflammation in the body. "Numerous studies have reported that eugenol possesses antibacterial, antiviral, antioxidant, anti-inflammatory, and analgesic effects. Eugenol has been widely used in dentistry to treat toothache and pulpitis. A previous study indicated that eugenol may be an ideal natural agent for use in oral care products."[258]

From toothaches to digestion and even infections, tarragon can be beneficial to the body and your food.

TEA TREE OIL

One of the most powerful essential oils, tea tree oil is used for many different things, from facial washes and shampoos to cleaning products for the home. It has antiseptic, antibacterial, and antifungal properties that are great for healing cuts and abrasions on the skin and help heal acne. Tea tree oil contains many compounds that can penetrate membranes and, therefore, kill bacteria and infections on the skin and in the air.

Do you have eczema or an itchy scalp? Tea tree oil can help reduce itching and swelling and may heal excessive dandruff related to dermatitis. Tea tree oil, or melaleuca, may also have anti-viral properties. One study explored the effects tea tree oil and eucalyptus oil has on the herpes virus and warts, and the results indicated that both TTO and EUO can exert a direct antiviral effect on HSV.[259]

The compound terpinen-4-ol in tea tree oil helps fight chronic inflammation. Tea tree oil may fight bacteria, even antibiotic-resistant strains like staph, which is the cause of illnesses such as UTIs, strep throat, sinus infections, and many more.[260] So when you have that nasty cough or experience a sinus infection, grab tea tree oil for faster relief.

Do you have halitosis? If you do, it's okay; relief is on the way! The antimicrobial properties in tea tree oil help fight against microbes and bacteria in the mouth, tongue, and throat, which is usually where bad breath comes from. Hate going to the dentist and hearing that two teeth must be pulled? What are you going to do? It is a great idea to use tea tree oil as a rinse or mouthwash to fight against infection and bad breath. Use it as a rinse; do not swallow. Not only will it help protect against bad breath and infection, it's anti-inflammatory properties will help with the swelling.

So remember, tea tree oil (melaleuca) can be used in the home to produce a calming effect and a pleasant aroma. And use it topically to fight off several infections and bacteria; just make sure you purchase the 100 percent natural essential oil.

THYME

Here we go, another herb … I am starting to think there's something to these herbs and their healing abilities. Thyme has antibacterial, antiseptic, and antifungal properties and has been used for medicinal purposes since ancient times, from healing a cut to preventing food poisoning. Did you know if you struggle with constipation or just want ease when using the restroom, thyme, as a natural diuretic, can be of assistance? Thyme is great for combating bacteria in two of the main places we experience several different strains of bacteria— our mouths and throats.[261] One study conducted at the U.S. Library of Medicine showed thyme oil demonstrated a good efficacy against antibiotic-resistant strains of 120 tested bacteria from patients. The results suggested that the oil from thyme exhibited strong activity against all the clinical strains.[262]

Thyme not only tastes great on food, but it helps prevent food contamination and reduce further contamination of already contaminated food. "The volatile oil components of thyme have also been shown to have antimicrobial activity against a host of different bacteria and fungi such as staphylococcus aureus, bacillus subtilis, Escherichia coli and shigella sonnei."[263]

Thyme may help reduce LDL or bad cholesterol and reduce triglyceride levels while increasing HDL or good cholesterol numbers. Also, thyme contains the phenol carvacrol,[264] which may fight cancer cells. From breast cancer to prostate and even lung cancer, carvacrol, in certain studies, has expedited cancer cell death without being toxic. Another study suggests that carvacrol may have therapeutic potential for the prevention and treatment of colon cancer.[265] Therefore, thyme and thyme oil may have antitumor properties and affects.

Thyme may make you feel better because, once again, the carvacrol it contains can affect the brain's neurotransmitters or waves that affect our serotonin levels and can improve our mood.[266]

I bet you didn't know thymol, the active ingredient in thyme, is used in mouthwash, and it helps clean bacteria in the mouth. Maybe the ancient people who cooked with herbs knew what they were doing.

TURMERIC

Often referred to as "liquid gold," turmeric has so many benefits, it's unbelievable. Did you know if you mix turmeric with a fat (I use almond milk), the combined bioactive properties have the same affects as pharmaceutical antibiotics on the body when ingested? Wow! Turmeric contains a compound called curcumin, which gives turmeric its antioxidant and medicinal properties. However, turmeric is not easily absorbed in the blood stream, so it is ideal to mix common pepper or piperine with it to improve the chances of absorption.[267]

Chronic inflammation is the root cause of several diseases such as heart disease, cancer, and high cholesterol. Curcumin is an anti-inflammatory and may help fight skin cancer.[268] One study from the National Institute of Health reported that curcumin inhibits NF-kappaB (a nuclear factor active in most cancers) and selectively induces apoptosis of melanoma cells but not normal melanocytes,[269] thus indicating its effects on reducing disease and inflammation.[270]

Have a big event coming up and trying to lose a few pounds, or do you suffer from metabolic syndrome or added adipose tissue around the stomach? Curcumin may help you lose weight and decrease body fat, especially in the midsection. A recent study showed that curcumin administration increased weight loss, enhanced the percentage of body fat reduction, increased waistline reduction, improved the reduction of hip circumference, and enhanced the reduction of BMI. It may be used to curb cravings and even decrease appetite.[271]

Sugar is one of the main causes of weight gain, and curcumin is great at balancing blood sugar levels for diabetics. It helps regulate blood sugar by changing how the glucose is metabolized in the body. Are you at risk for atherosclerosis? Do you have high cholesterol? Turmeric, when taken in the capsule form, may inhibit oxidation of low-density lipoproteins or LDL cholesterol. One study showed improved endothelial function, a decrease in bad cholesterol and an improvement in cholesterol levels, making it ideal for combating atherosclerosis or hardening of the arteries.[272]

Anxiety and depression are on the rise as our jobs and families require more time and daily attention. Thousands of people take antidepressants to help them cope, but curcumin found in turmeric may help. It may help boost serotonin levels in the brain,[273] and after a study was conducted for six weeks, it showed the ability to improve depression symptoms and boost the neurotrophic factor (linked to the cause of depression in the brain when low) levels in the brain.[274]

From arthritis to weight loss, cognitive health, and high cholesterol, turmeric is an all-around beneficial spice. I see why Indians eat so much curry and have used it medicinally for centuries.

THIAMINE

It is a vitamin but not just any vitamin; thiamine is vitamin B1, which is necessary for the body to convert carbohydrates to energy. Thiamine is found in foods, but since it's a water-soluble vitamin, once its cooked, the nutrient is destroyed and comes out in the water the food was cooked in. B1 can often be purchased in the pill form to make sure you're getting in adequate amounts to help prevent deficiency. Thiamin can be used to help reduce inflammation and improve athletic ability. B1 vitamin is essential to the flow of electrolytes throughout the body and cells.[275]

Furthermore, B vitamins are great for pregnant women and necessary even when your body is under stress because it helps combat tension on the body.

You can get thiamine through food, and that is ideally the way you should get all your vitamins; however, if you're not eating enough raw fruits and vegetables, supplementing with a vitamin is great as well.

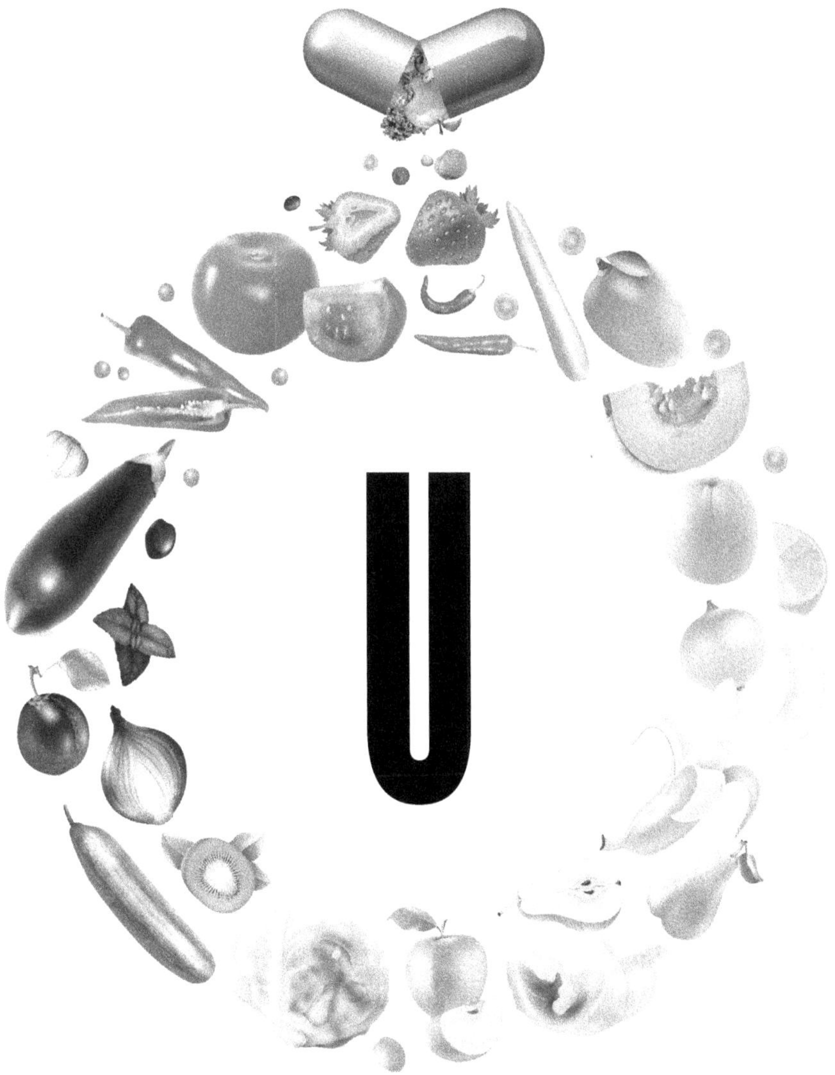
U

U GLI FRUIT

Yes, you read that correctly—ugly fruit. Granted, there is nothing ugly about this fruit; it is beautiful in appearance and the benefits to the body. It's a citrus fruit native to Jamaica, packed with calcium and vitamin C, with a sweet yet tangy taste. One of the key benefits of ugli fruit is that it helps with weight loss. *How?* It's low in calories and full of fiber, which helps to keep you fuller longer, preventing overeating and the digestion of unwanted toxins in the body. It contains no carbohydrates, no fat, and will even give you a boost of energy before a workout. Fiber is also good for the heart, and ugli fruit contains pectin,[276] which is a plant-based fiber that helps lower cholesterol and is great for digestion. Lower cholesterol levels and low triglycerides aids in reducing the risk of developing heart disease or hypertension. Also, since ugli fruit is low in calories with no carbs, it is a good option for people with diabetes. It helps balance and maintain low blood sugar levels and falls low on the glycemic index, which is great for those who have a family history of type 2 diabetes.

Ugli fruit's pectin slows down the activity of enzymes that break down starches and sugar in the digestive system, helping to protect against spikes in blood sugar, and it slows the absorption of sugar and carbohydrates.

Like most citrus fruits, ugli fruit helps your immune system. The high amount of vitamin C and other antioxidants helps you fight off infections and prevents the replication of further illness. It aids in fighting the free radical damage we get from our diets and the environment and boosts the white blood cell count, the cells that fight off infections. It has more than sixty percent of the RDA of vitamins in just half the fruit, so consuming one a day is a great addition to your routine. Even though the name is "ugli fruit," it is beautiful on the inside and will make us healthy and beautiful on the inside as well.

USNEA

Usnea is a lichen similar to algae and fungus. It's native to the Chinese culture and has been used to treat conditions for years. Do you suffer from a weak immune system like me or experience urinary tract infections often? Usnea is used to aid in secretion production to help remove toxins from the kidneys and filter the urinary tract. It's used to help balance the microbial system in the gut and digestive system while improving the immune system and the mucus membranes.

Usnea has antibacterial and antiviral properties, and it can kill harmful bacteria while maintaining healthy bacteria. Also, it helps to rid the body of unwanted viruses and promotes a healthy system. Whether it be a weakened immune system, an open wound or abrasion, herpes, strep throat, or even a respiratory infection, usnea is the herb to turn to for relief.

Usnea may also aid in weight loss and help treat and improve the appearance of sores from human papilloma virus (HPV), according to webmd.com. You can choose to take usnea in the capsule, powder, or tea form, and you'll find it at your nearest grocery store.

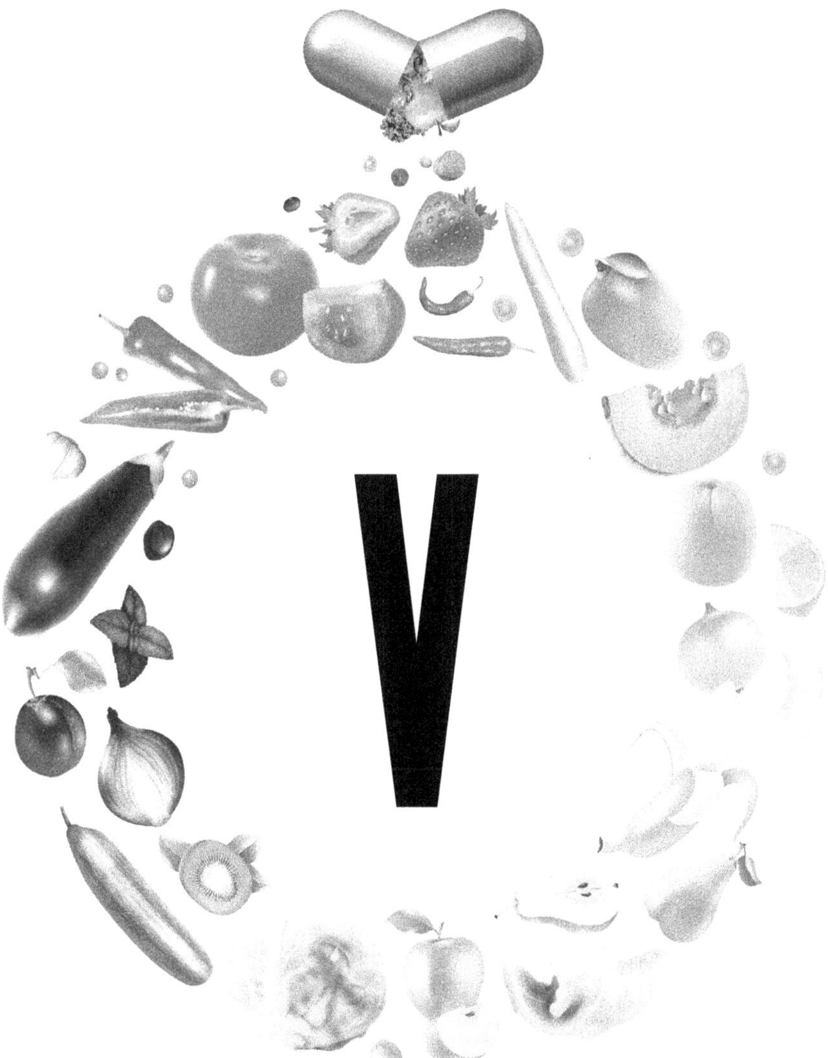

VANILLA OIL

Used when baking to give desserts that extra flavor, vanilla oil can be used for aromatherapy in the home, too. Vanilla is a great fragrant and good for flavoring, but it also provides excellent health benefits. Do you suffer from erectile dysfunction or struggle with sexual arousal? Vanilla can help boost the natural libido and enhance hormone levels. Did you know vanilla oil is so calming and relaxing that it's considered a sedative? That means relief at last for us women when it comes to our cycle! Vanilla oil can help relieve the pain and cramping we experience during our periods and ease our mood swings as well.

Vanilla is packed with antioxidants that help fight free radical damage and fight against some of the most common diseases we face. According to a study published in the *Journal of Agricultural* and *Food Chemistry,* pure vanilla extract, made with cured vanilla beans and sixty percent aqueous ethyl alcohol, has high levels of antioxidant activity. The study noted that the results point toward the potential use of vanilla extract components as antioxidants for food preservation and in health supplements as nutraceuticals.[277]

Vanilla oil may be used to help fight infections and even combat cancer and cancer cells because it inhibits the growth of the cells by preventing the cells' oxidation. As a calming agent, vanilla oil can help with high blood pressure and aid in depression and anxiety. It sends a soothing signal to the brain and calms the muscles and the entire body. Finally, a calm body will help fight inflammation because inflammation is a cause of stress on the body. Anti-inflammatory foods help with every bodily system and fight conditions and diseases caused by inflammation such as edema.

Whether you use vanilla to add flavor to your favorite cake, enhance your home's aroma, or decrease depression symptoms, vanilla is a great asset to have around.

VERBENA

It can be used as a tea and it's considered an herb. Lemon verbena has several uses, but it is mainly used to help relieve stomach and digestive issues. It is native to South America and thrives in warm climates. Lemon verbena may fight staph infections, which is one of the hardest infections to fight because of its resistance to antibiotics. According to a recent study, "An ethanolic extract of lemon verbena can prevent the growth of staphylococcus aureus."[278]

Furthermore, verbena can help repair and aid in muscle growth by protecting white blood cells against oxidative damage. As we know, inflammation is one of the leading causes of several diseases. Lemon verbena may fight chronic inflammation.

You may struggle to find lemon verbena at your local grocery store, but you can grow it in your own garden. Just purchase the seeds and put them in a pot. Remember, it likes warm climates, so be sure to bring the plant inside if the weather turns cold. Use the herb in your desserts, teas, and even as a pleasant aroma in your home.

VALERIAN ROOT

Many people often overlook this herb, most likely because they're unaware of its benefits, so it's commonly swapped for melatonin. Valerian root has a profound effect on sleep. If you ever purchase yogi tea or another brand of medicinal teas, look on the back of their "sleepy time" tea package, and you may see valerian root listed in the ingredients. It can help with insomnia because it not only helps you get to sleep, but it enhances your overall quality of sleep.

This root contains compounds and antioxidants that can affect the brain, increasing the brain's GABA (Gamma Amino- butyric acid) levels and acting as a natural sedative. Did you just switch to a new job or change roles at your current job? Do you get easily overwhelmed and anxious like me? If so, it can cause stress and anxiety on the body and brain. However, valerian root can increase the amount of GABA through GABA receptors, which will help regulate nerve cells and calm anxiety, acting as an antidepressant.[279]

When your body is calm, you have less internal stress, which is helpful to your major organs, especially your heart. Chronic stress can be detrimental to your health, and some have developed ulcers due to high levels of stress. It is important to know how to properly manage your stress, and valerian root is a great addition. So it's not a shocker that valerian root may help reduce your blood pressure and improve overall heart health.

Ladies, this one is for you: Valerian root helps the body calm itself, including when we have our monthly menstrual visit. If you suffer from severe cramps, upset stomach, or excessive anxiety during that time, valerian root relaxes the muscles, decreases the uterus contractions, and can even keep us calm, instead of yelling at our significant others. Truly a blessing for all.

Remember not to take multiple sleep aids together. Whether you choose melatonin or valerian root, make sure you're getting the relief you need.

HEALTH AND HAPPINESS

Some people are naturally thin because of genetics, while others struggle with their weight; it's just a fact of life. My brother didn't necessarily struggle with his weight; we just considered him "big boned," but he was overweight, and he didn't realize it until he was in his early twenties. My cousin, who is naturally thin, asked him, "Are you happy with yourself, with the way you look when you look in the mirror?" My brother couldn't respond, and he thought long and hard about that question. Two days later, he decided to make a change. He was never diagnosed with any health problems besides asthma, which he was born with, but he wasn't happy with his appearance. He cut out all fast food and drinks besides water. He worked out five days a week religiously and stopped eating after eight p.m. He lost sixty pounds, his asthma improved so much that he doesn't even use his inhaler, and he has more self-confidence. He later thanked his cousin for making him realize he wasn't happy with himself and he needed to make a change before it was too late.

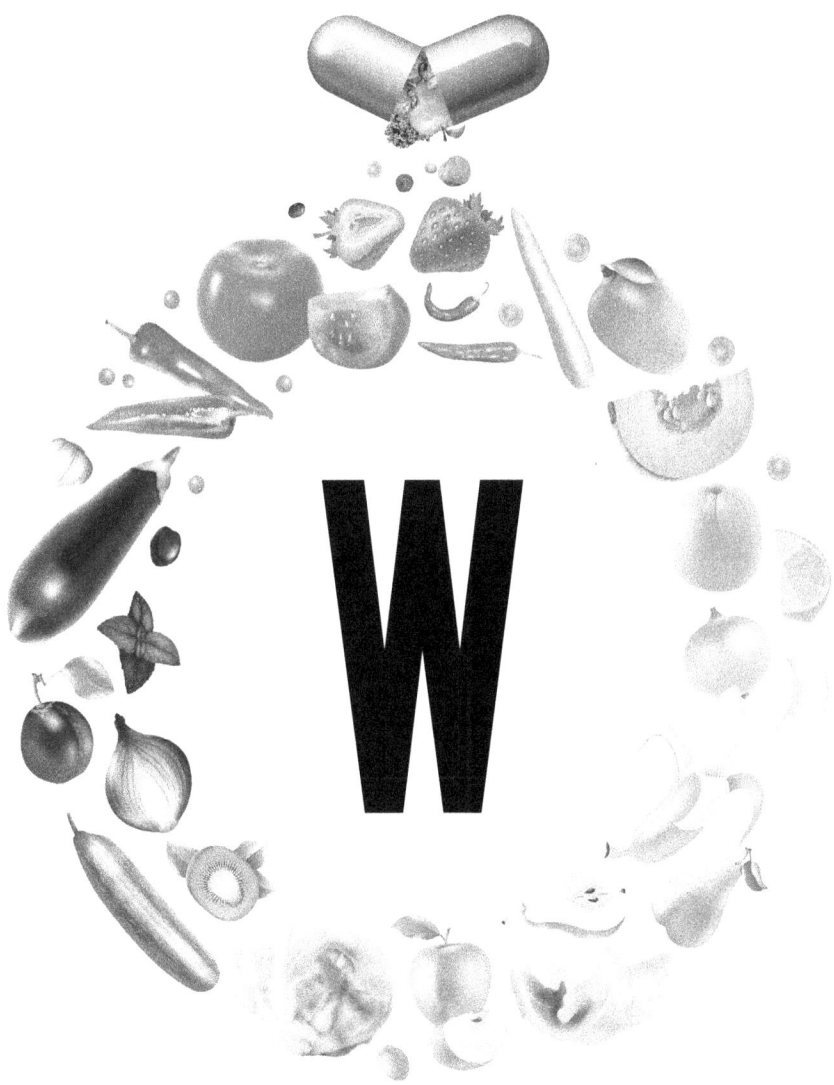

WATERMELON

Known as a refreshing summer treat, watermelon is packed with lots of nutrients, vitamins, and water. Watermelon isn't just a summertime fruit; it has a load of benefits essential for the body, and we will discuss a few here.

Did you know watermelon originated in Africa, and there are more than 1000 varieties of watermelon, even a yellow one? Watermelon contains a great deal of vitamin C and vitamin A along with antioxidants to aid in an excellent immune system and great health. It helps fight off free radical damage and decrease unwanted inflammation in the body.

Ever wonder how to manage your high blood pressure? Just eat some watermelon; it contains an amino acid called arginine, which has been known to help improve blood flow in the heart and synthesize nitric oxide, thus keeping the blood moving efficiently in the heart and throughout the body. Furthermore, watermelon contains about ten percent of your daily value of potassium and magnesium, aiding in reducing high blood pressure the natural way and decreasing your chances of developing a stroke or heart disease.[280]

Did you know watermelon contains lycopene? *Great, what does that have to do with me?* Lycopene is a compound found in many fruits that gives them their pigment or color. However, lycopene may help reduce inflammation and improve your cholesterol, and since it acts as an antioxidant, it even protects your cells from damage. Ever wonder why watermelon is so refreshing? Well it's mostly made of water (hence the name). Packed with water, watermelon aids in dehydration and helps remove unwanted toxins, waste, and it assists with water retention or edema by helping to flush the body system. Furthermore, the potassium watermelon contains acts as an electrolyte, giving your body hydration balance, improving circulation and boosting oxygen through the body. Trying to drop a few pounds? Watermelon has your back. Packed with vitamins and nutrients as well as water, it helps you feel fuller longer, assisting in a decreased appetite all while relieving any symptoms of stomach pain or bloating. That's great for us women during that time of the month. Now, we discussed how watermelon is great during the summer because it gives you hydration on those hot days, but when you're outside burning up in the heat, what about your skin? Watermelon helps with that, too! Because it's full of vitamin C and A, watermelon increases collagen production in the skin, decreasing wrinkles and aiding in improved elasticity, protecting the skin against sun damage. Furthermore, the vitamin A can help by keeping the healthy skin cells we have intact and preventing any further damage. Watermelon's vitamin A is also great for the eyes. It helps fight against macular degeneration and, in turn, helps prevent cornea damage and even blindness.

Are you frequently burping or feel a burning sensation in your throat? Have you ever been diagnosed with GERD or acid reflux? Watermelon can help relieve some of your pain and symptoms. It is believed to help soothe the gastrointestinal tract and reduce inflammation all while aiding in bringing the body's pH levels back into balance, decreasing any elevated acid levels.

Watermelon can improve your kidney function by removing unwanted toxins and filtering the body since it is a natural diuretic. Do you workout hard like me, and you're always looking for some form of relief for your sore muscles? Watermelon is great for muscle recovery. The potassium it contains helps relieve sore muscles and prevents cramps because it balances your potassium and sodium levels. It's great for repairing damage to the tendons and ligaments with its vitamin C. Trust me, I know from experience. When I tore my LCL, watermelon helped me tremendously in my recovery.

Watermelon comes in many different colors, shapes, and sizes, but they can all benefit you!

WILLOW BARK

Is it part of a tree, or is it a plant? Actually, willow bark comes from several different types of trees and is used to make medicine. It may be used to treat pain from cramps, Charlie horses, and joint pain. *How does the bark help ease the pain?* Willow bark contains salicin, a compound that acts as an anti-inflammatory in the body. The body responds to it like aspirin.[281] As an anti-inflammatory, willow bark may help relieve back pain, severe muscle aches, and even help treat a cold.

You can purchase willow bark at your local health food store in the capsule, liquid, or tea form.

WHEAT BRAN

I eat a lot of wheat. This is like wheat germ, right? Wrong. Wheat bran is the outside part of the wheat kernel. It is full of fiber and nutrients, and it looks like small light brown flakes. One key benefit of wheat bran is that it can help with regularity by pushing out unwanted toxins and stool because it's an insoluble fiber. It contains more than six grams of fiber in just one-fourth cup, so you can easily sprinkle it on top of your oatmeal for added fiber, and it's a good source of protein. Wheat bran is also beneficial if you suffer from constipation, diverticulitis, or bloating because it improves good gut bacteria and eases stomach pain, riding you of unnecessary waste. Furthermore, wheat bran acts as a prebiotic, remaining undigested in the gut, thus becoming a source for fuel and a nutrient for the gut. You know getting rid of unnecessary waste and toxins makes you feel lighter; well, that's because you *are* lighter. Wheat bran aids in weight loss because it makes you feel fuller longer, so throughout the day, you eat less and lose weight.

Lastly, wheat bran contains a lot of minerals and nutrients such as manganese, folate, and selenium, and these nutrients are great for absorption, proper bone development, and strengthening the immune system. Whether you choose to add wheat bran to your morning smoothie, in your baked goods, or on top of your oatmeal, your body will be happy, and your gut will feel great.

WHEATGRASS

It is a grass—literally a grass. Usually blended in a shot or a powder, wheatgrass is packed with chlorophyll, which gives it its green color and antioxidants. Wheatgrass is considered a superfood because it is *that* beneficial to your body. From fighting off infections, alkalizing your body, improving skin irritations like psoriasis, to helping to balance your sugar levels, wheatgrass is a must have in the diet. Let's dig a little deeper into a few health benefits. I can't mention them all, or you'll be reading for days!

Wheatgrass may improve overall cholesterol levels and help prevent hyperlipidemia. According to a study by the National Institute of Health, wheatgrass supplementation with a high-fat diet resulted in improved lipid levels, significantly reduced MDA levels, and increased GSH and vitamin C levels, indicating the beneficial role of wheatgrass in improving hyperlipidemia and oxidative stress.[282] Wheatgrass is also beneficial in helping to reduce excessive inflammation in the body and fighting against diseases normally caused by oxidative stress and free radical damage.

Have you ever eaten a lot of iron or drank a lot of Gatorade to get electrolytes but still feel tired? It's not just in your head; you may have a problem with absorption. Wheatgrass helps alkalize the body and improve absorption, so when you ingest things, your body can get the full benefits and nutrients it deserves. As Americans, we eat way too much fast food, which creates an unhealthy body system and gut, making us more at risk for developing cancers and other chronic diseases. Wheatgrass naturally helps balance our bodies' pH levels and ultimately fights against acidosis because of the amount of chlorophyll it contains. Acidosis occurs when your body's fluid contains too much acid.[283]

Ultimately, wheatgrass is a tremendous health benefit to us. It can help improve sleep, it's a natural antibacterial, it balances hormones, and helps you lose weight. Now remember, wheatgrass is still a grass, so it has an earthy taste, and it may take some time to adjust to your palate, but it is definitely worth the effort and adjustment to your overall health. You can purchase it at your local health food store, and they will blend it for you.

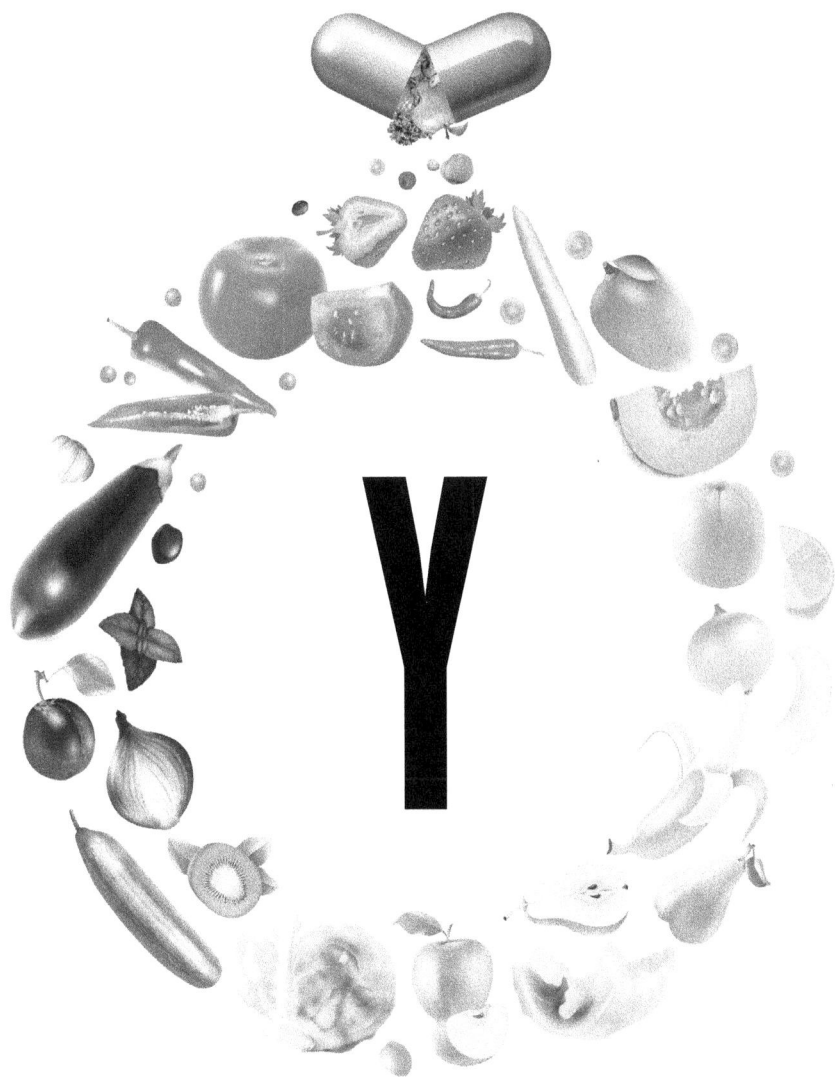

YOGURT

I usually add cinnamon, berries, and a little stevia to my yogurt. Some people add it to their smoothies for added protein and to make them creamy. Others even use Greek yogurt as a substitute for sour cream. Yogurt is a creamy dairy product fermented to make it smooth and rich. It's considered a probiotic, and it's packed with protein. Probiotics are live bacteria or microorganisms known to promote healthy gut bacteria. However, yogurt is not just beneficial for the gut; it can also help with the heart, blood pressure, and immune system, just to name a few. Let's look a little closer at the different types of yogurt and how it can help us.

The top benefit for yogurt is that it helps with digestive issues in the stomach. Whether you have experienced IBS, constipation, or just an upset stomach, the healthy bacteria yogurt has may help soothe the digestive tract and provide comfort. Yogurt also helps with absorption and digestion, which, in turn, may help regulate your blood sugar and decrease the chances of developing type 2 diabetes.

As women, we are at a higher risk for developing osteopenia or osteoporosis as we age; however, eating foods packed with calcium and vitamin D can help aid in maintaining strong bones. Yogurt is full of calcium, and vitamin D is usually added, which will help support bone mass and decrease bone loss while strengthening our bones. Looking to drop a few pounds or control your sugar intake? Yogurt may help you by increasing fat loss, and the protein it contains will keep you fuller longer, resulting in a decreased intake of food throughout the day. On the other hand, yogurt helps keep you from getting sick regularly by boosting your immune system to fight off unwanted germs and bacteria. Yogurt's probiotics help with immune function by increasing cytokine-producing cells in the intestines and fighting against immune mediated diseases such as the flu, the common cold, or fever.

I mentioned that yogurt is good for the heart and regulating blood pressure, but how? Yogurt is packed with potassium, and we all know by now that it's important to have a good potassium/sodium balance in the body. "Potassium is believed to help decrease sodium re-absorption and alter nervous system cell function to help reduce blood pressure and improve heart health."[284]

Yogurt is perfect for individuals who have recently taken some form of medicine or antibiotics because antibiotics kill both good and bad bacteria. Yogurt helps replace the good bacteria that was destroyed. Just remember a few things when purchasing yogurt: It is best to purchase raw yogurt from goats or sheep. Buy plain yogurt and add your own flavoring or sugar if desired. Greek yogurt is packed with protein, and it's a great substitute for higher fat dairy products. Just make sure it's strained. You can purchase yogurt at your local grocery or convenience store. Enjoy it regularly.

YUCCA

Often substituted for potato, yucca has a stringy texture similar to pumpkin. It's a root vegetable and can be made into fries or tortillas or added to your favorite dish for a thicker and richer texture. Yucca root is from South America and has been known to help lower sugar levels and fight against oxidative stress. It is a high-carb and high-calorie food, but it's full of fiber and vitamin C. Yucca is considered low on the glycemic index, so it is a great carb for those who are watching their sugar levels and better for you than some carbs that will cause a spike. However, yucca root is high in antioxidants which helps us not only fight off unwanted bacteria and resist oxidative stress, but it also helps us stay healthy by riding us of harmful viruses and fungi that normally lead to infections.

Do you suffer from dark spots or hyperpigmentation like me? Usually, it's due to an inadequate intake of vitamin C. I'm allergic to citrus fruits, which normally contain the highest amounts of vitamin C. Go figure, right? However, yucca root is full of vitamin C. which not only aids in exfoliating the skin and eliminating dead skin cells, but it also helps brighten the skin and give a youthful glow because of the collagen synthesis that vitamin C promotes.

Yucca root may help with arthritis pain and stiffness. It contains manganese, a mineral that is important for proper body function. According to a study recorded by the U.S. National Library of Medicine, women from the ages of fifty-five to fifty-nine who took manganese had a lower risk of rheumatoid arthritis and joint pain. Yucca's antioxidants also help reduce inflammation on the joints.[285]

Yucca has a dark brown exterior and a white or tan interior, and it's usually long and thin. It's found next to other root vegetables or exotic foods.

YERBA SANTA

What is that? Yerba santa is a leaf traditionally used to make medicine. It can be used to relive a cough, infections, joint pain, and even fever or dry mouth. Have severe constipation or a bruise? When placed inside a warm towel, yerba santa can relieve the tension of a bruise, and it's also a natural tonic. For congestion, yerba santa contains properties that loosen phlegm in the sinuses and chest. You can purchase this herb in the vitamin form at your local health food store.

YARROW

Is it a vegetable or an herb? Yarrow is similar in appearance to chamomile and is known to help fight inflammation and even has antibacterial properties. Previously, some cultures ingested parts of the herb in several dishes. However, yarrow is great for cuts and bruises and has several other medicinal purposes. The herb contains the alkaloid achilleine, which helps wounds heal by encouraging blood clotting. It can also aid in fighting infections because it's a natural antiseptic. If you have eczema or atopic dermatitis like me, you're probably always looking for relief from the pain and itching. Yarrow is the answer. According to a study done by the National Institute of Health, yarrow showed anti-inflammatory properties related to the content of flavonoids and sesquiterpene lactones in the raw material it contains.[286]

Yarrow's anti-inflammatory properties work great for the intestines, gastrointestinal tract, and the reproductive organs to help fight issues. Speaking of reproductive organs, yarrow also provides aid to nursing mothers who suffer from tender nipples or mastitis.[287] Mastitis is inflammation of the mammary gland in the breast or udder, typically due to a bacterial infection via a damaged nipple or teat. Yarrow relieves the inflammation and tenderness and even fights the infection while healing the nipples and improving circulation.[288]

You can use the leaves and the stems to aid in relieving health concerns and cooking. Purchase yarrow at your local plant store or farmers market.

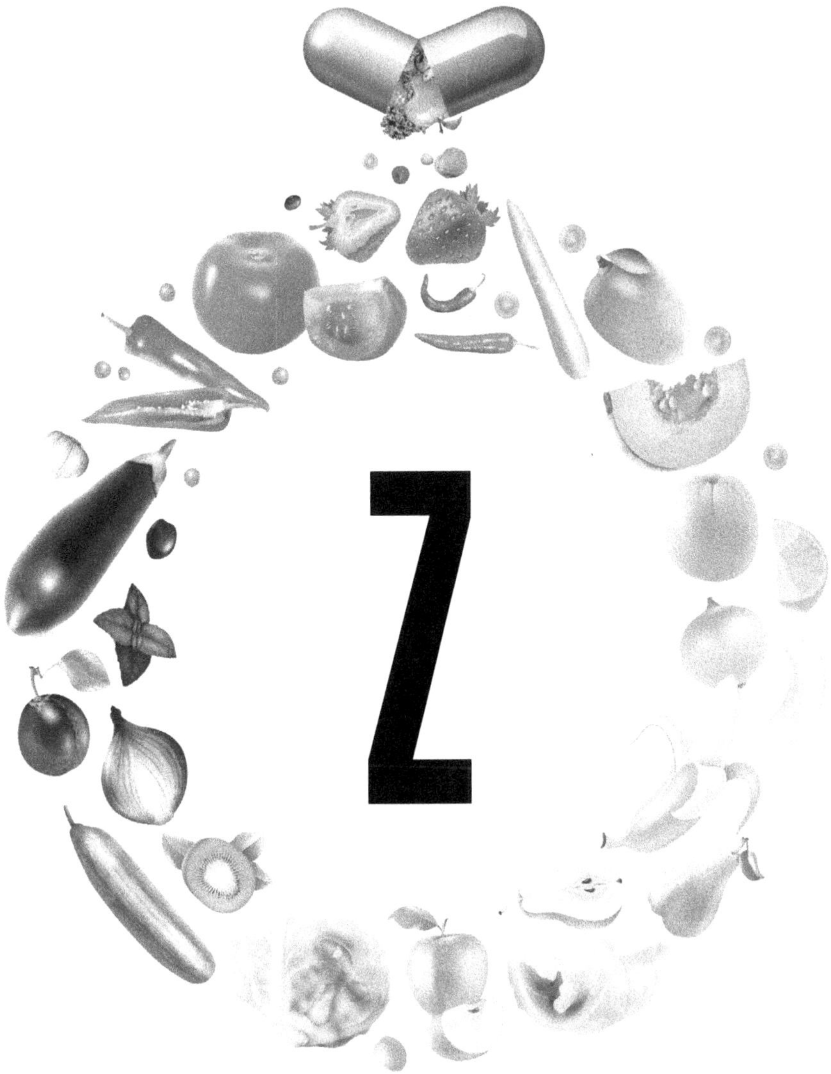
Z

ZUCCHINI

Often paired with its partner, squash, zucchini is a low-calorie, versatile vegetable packed with several nutrients. Now trending due to its ability to replace common carbohydrates, zucchini can be a great base to your favorite meal, especially if you're eating low carbs or trying to lose weight. Zucchini is full of antioxidants and compounds that are great for everyone, even diabetics, since it's low on the glycemic index. It's considered a summer squash and has high water content, making it ideal for removal of toxins.[289]

Zucchini's antioxidants can help fight inflammation, boost your immune system to fight off infection and help combat heart disease and free radical damage due to oxidative stress. Most of the nutrients are in the skin of zucchini; therefore, it's best not to peel it. The seeds contain phytonutrients that may help with plaque buildup in the arteries and improve the cardiovascular and digestive systems. So if you suffer from constipation or IBS, zucchini may help improve your symptoms.[290]

High cholesterol or high blood pressure? Zucchini contains a fiber called pectin that may naturally help lower cholesterol, and since most of us Americans eat too much sodium, the potassium it contains helps balance our sodium/potassium levels, which helps prevent heart disease and/or stroke.[291]

Pregnant or an athlete? Zucchini contains folate and B vitamins that are perfect for expecting moms because folate helps with cell development, fights against neural tube defects, and helps the body synthesize DNA to properly create new life. Also, its B vitamins help improve metabolism, boost energy, and it helps fire the synapses in the brain.[292]

Earlier, we learned that lutein and zeaxanthin are compounds that improve the eye function and maintain proper health, but how? They block UV rays and damage caused by free radicals in the environment and protect the eye tissue, aiding in the prevention of eye diseases such as macular degeneration and glaucoma.[293]

Remember, zucchini may help you lose weight due to its high water content, low calories, low carbohydrates, and high fiber, helping you feel fuller longer and riding the body of useless toxins. It is ideal to eat the entire vegetable with the skin and seeds, or mix it with other foods if you aren't a fan of the bitter taste.

JUST WHAT THE DOCTOR DIDN'T ORDER

When my aunt turned sixty years old, she began developing health problems. Initially, she thought she had bad heart burn or even acid reflux, so she went to her primary care physician to find out what was wrong. The doctor prescribed her Prilosec OTC and directed her to also take an anti-inflammatory daily. She was in severe pain and experienced bad side effects from the medication, so she reached out to me for help. I told her she may have GERD but to ask for a second opinion for a proper diagnosis. She went to an ear and throat doctor, and he told her she did, indeed, have GERD. She came back to me and asked what would help her instead of medication. I advised her to drink aloe vera juice and avoid acid foods like tomatoes. She no longer has any pain, her GERD is nonexistent, and the inflammation has decreased. She has more energy, she stopped the medication months ago, and she's healthier overall. When she went back to her PCP, he even asked her what she did to improve so quickly, and she told him she healed herself naturally.

START *REALLY* LIVING!

Whether you read this book cover to cover, only one chapter, or skimmed through, I hope this information not only educated you on the importance of real food and how it can benefit you, but also helped you see that food is not meant to only satisfy our palates; it also heals. Our bodies are amazing, from what they can handle to how they fight disease and infections, and by choosing to make wise food choices, you may vastly improve your health. Implementing healthy foods into your daily regimen will decrease your chances of developing health problems long term and, ultimately, help break unhealthy generational food habits. You may choose to continue to take medication while adding healthier food options to your diet or heal solely with food. Either way, you can now enjoy real food and start *really* living with *The Edible Cure*.

ACKNOWLEDGMENTS

Writing a book was more challenging yet rewarding than I could have ever imagined. I want to thank my parents, Kathy and Rickey Grant, for always inspiring and motivating me to reach for the stars and fulfill my dreams. Your expectations and determination motivated me to never give up and keep going, even when things got rough.

I am grateful to one of my best friends, Bryan Pitts. You asked me weekly how the book was coming, and even when I wanted to quit, you told me, "You're going to finish this book, come what may!" You are an excellent example of what friends are supposed to do to support each other.

A very special thanks to Christopher Smoot Jr., who was there from the beginning and told me, "You can do anything you set your mind to, so if you want to write a book, do it!" You listened to me complain at night and heard my frustrations about how much further I wanted to be in the book; you even helped me revise different sections to sound more fluid. I do not know if I would have been able to complete this book without you. I am forever indebted to you.

To my only brother, Rickey Grant Jr., thank you for inspiring me to write this book to help others, especially after seeing the changes you made to your diet and lifestyle. You not only helped me see the bigger picture, but you also assisted me in coming up with the style and structure of the book. Even when we talked daily about my work struggles, you continued to motivate me to find energy and dig deep to work on my passion.

To Angelica Vaughan, I appreciate you always finding a way to make me laugh when I was stressed out and giving me joy to keep going so I could pursue my dream of completing the book. Thank you for listening to me vent and telling me, "Sis, you got this. I know you; keep pushing." You had more faith in me than I had in myself, and it was just the boost I needed.

To Cameron J. Whitaker, sir we have known each other so long, and you have always inspired me to do better and be better. I appreciate you telling me, "It may take you several years, but just finish it out." That pushed me and showed me I could do this, even though I didn't believe it myself. Thank you for your encouragement, love, tough criticism, and support over the years to help me be a better person and now writer. You saw the good in me years ago, and now, I see it in myself, and I wouldn't be the woman I am today if it weren't for you, a true and genuine friend.

Thank you to all my family and friends who stuck by me through this process and even encouraged me to keep going. You are truly loved and valued.

Last but not least, thank you to my tribe, my readers, for purchasing this book and believing in my message enough to read it. If it weren't for you all, I would not have an audience. You all are greatly appreciated, and I hope I can continue to inspire you the way you inspire me.

Thank you for reading *The Edible Cure*
If you enjoyed this book or found it useful,
please leave an online review.

KEEP IN TOUCH WITH KRISTINA GRANT

Website: www.igrantunutrition.com
Facebook: IgrantuNutrition
Instagram: @igrantu & @granted_wellness

NOTES

1   LLC, Webmd, "PECTIN" https://www.webmd.com, https://www.webmd.com/vitamins/ai/ingredientmono-500/pectin (2019 June 6)

2   Carr AC, Maggini S. "Vitamin C and Immune Function," https://www.ncbi.nlm.nih.gov, https://www.ncbi.nlm.nih.gov/pubmed/29099763, (2018 September 30)

3   López Ledesma R.," Monounsaturated fatty acid (avocado) rich diet for mild hypercholesterolemia," https://www.ncbi.nlm.nih.gov/, https://www.ncbi.nlm.nih.gov/pubmed/8987188, (2019 Aug 11)

4   Johnson EJ., "The role of carotenoids in human health," https://www.ncbi.nlm.nih.gov/, https://www.ncbi.nlm.nih.gov/pubmed/12134711, (2019 Aug 10)

5   Shishehbor F, Mansoori A, Sarkaki AR, Jalali MT, Latifi SM, "Apple cider vinegar attenuates lipid profile in normal and diabetic rats," https://www.ncbi.nlm.nih.gov/, https://www.ncbi.nlm.nih.gov/pubmed/19630216, (2019, May 22)

6   Kondo T, Kishi M, Fushimi T, Ugajin S, Kaga T., "Vinegar intake reduces body weight, body fat mass, and serum triglyceride levels in obese Japanese subjects," https://www.ncbi.nlm.nih.gov/, https://www.ncbi.nlm.nih.gov/pubmed/19661687, (2019 May 17)

7   Kondo S, Tayama K, Tsukamoto Y, Ikeda K, Yamori Y., "Antihypertensive effects of acetic acid and vinegar on spontaneously hypertensive rats," https://www.ncbi.nlm.nih.gov/, https://www.ncbi.nlm.nih.gov/pubmed/11826965, (2019 May 22)

8   Sachdeva S., "Lactic acid peeling in superficial acne scarring in Indian skin," https://www.ncbi.nlm.nih.gov/, https://www.ncbi.nlm.nih.gov/pubmed/20883299, (2019 May 22)

9   Johnston CS, Buller AJ, "Vinegar and peanut products as complementary foods to reduce postprandial glycemia," https://www.ncbi.nlm.nih.gov/, https://www.ncbi.nlm.nih.gov/pubmed/16321601, (2019 May 19)

[10]   MD Jr Shiel, William C., "Peripheral Neuropathy," www.medicinenet.com, https://www.medicinenet.com/peripheral_neuropathy/article.htm, (2019 February 28)

[11]   Dawid-Pać R., "Medicinal plants used in treatment of inflammatory skin diseases," https://www.ncbi.nlm.nih.gov, https://www.ncbi.nlm.nih.gov/pmc/articles/PMC3834722/, (2019 March 12)

[12]   D'Antuono I, Carola A, Sena LM, Linsalata V, Cardinali A, Logrieco AF, Colucci MG, Apone F., "Artichoke Polyphenols Produce Skin Anti-Age Effects by Improving Endothelial Cell Integrity and Functionality," https://www.ncbi.nlm.nih.gov/, https://www.ncbi.nlm.nih.gov/pmc/articles/PMC6278506/, (2019 May 19)

[13]   Boots AW, Haenen GR, Bast A., "Health effects of quercetin: from antioxidant to nutraceutical," https://www.ncbi.nlm.nih.gov, https://www.ncbi.nlm.nih.gov/pubmed/18417116, (2018 March 13)

[14]   Mileo AM, Di Venere D, Linsalata V, Fraioli R, Miccadei S., "Artichoke polyphenols induce apoptosis and decrease the invasive potential of the human breast cancer cell line MDA-MB231," https://www.ncbi.nlm.nih.gov/, https://www.ncbi.nlm.nih.gov/pubmed/22170094, (2019 May 20)

[15]   Mileo AM, Di Venere D, Abbruzzese C, Miccadei S., "Long Term Exposure to Polyphenols of Artichoke (Cynara scolymus L.) Exerts Induction of Senescence Driven Growth Arrest in the MDA-MB231 Human Breast Cancer Cell Line," https://www.ncbi.nlm.nih.gov/, https://www.ncbi.nlm.nih.gov/pubmed/26180585, (2019 May 22)

[16]   Rondanelli M, Monteferrario F, Perna S, Faliva MA, Opizzi A., "Health-promoting properties of artichoke in preventing cardiovascular disease by its lipidic and glycemic-reducing action," https://www.ncbi.nlm.nih.gov/, https://www.ncbi.nlm.nih.gov/pubmed/23923586, (2019 May 22)

[17]   Santos HO, Bueno AA, Mota JF, "The effect of artichoke on lipid profile: A review of possible mechanisms of action," https://www.ncbi.nlm.nih.gov/, https://www.ncbi.nlm.nih.gov/pubmed/30308247, (2019 May 22)

[18]   Ertesvag A, Engedal N, Naderi S, Blomhoff HK., "Retinoic acid stimulates the cell cycle machinery in normal T cells: involvement of retinoic acid receptor-mediated IL-2 secretion," https://www.ncbi.nlm.nih.gov, https://www.ncbi.nlm.nih.gov/pubmed/12421932, (2018 September 30)

[19] Mahboubi M., "Natural therapeutic approach of Nigella sativa (Black seed) fixed oil in management of Sinusitis," https://www.ncbi.nlm.nih.gov, https://www.ncbi.nlm.nih.gov/pmc/articles/PMC5884000/, (2019 October 11)

[20] Ivankovic S., Stojkovic R., Jukic M., Milos M., Milos M., Jurin M.,, "The antitumor activity of thymoquinone and thymohydroquinone in vitro and in vivo," https://www.ncbi.nlm.nih.gov, https://www.ncbi.nlm.nih.gov/pubmed/17080016, (2019 October 11)

[21] STECKO, KATARZYNA, "An Herbal Extract Inhibits the Development of Pancreatic Cancer," http://www.clinicaleducation.org, http://www.clinicaleducation.org/resources/abstracts/an-herbal-extract-inhibits-the-development-of-pancreatic-cancer/, (2019 October 11)

[22] Yousefi M., Barikbin B., Kamalinejad M., Abolhasani E., Ebadi A., Younespour S., Manouchehrian M., Hejazi S., "Comparison of therapeutic effect of topical Nigella with Betamethasone and Eucerin in hand eczema," https://www.ncbi.nlm.nih.gov, https://www.ncbi.nlm.nih.gov/pubmed/23198836, (2019 October 11)

[23] Murli L. Mathur, Jyoti Gaur, Ruchika Sharma, Kripa Ram Haldiya, "Antidiabetic Properties of a Spice Plant *Nigella sativa,*" https://www.jofem.org, https://www.jofem.org/index.php/jofem/article/viewArticle/15/15, (2019 October 11)

[24] Karkala, Pooja, https://www.stylecraze.com. https://www.stylecraze.com/articles/how-to-use-kalonji-black-seed-oil-for-hair-growth-baldness/#gref, (2019 October 11)

[25] Kolahdooz M, Nasri S, Modarres SZ, Kianbakht S, Huseini HF, "Effects of Nigella sativa L. seed oil on abnormal semen quality in infertile men: a randomized, double-blind, placebo-controlled clinical trial," https://www.ncbi.nlm.nih.gov, https://www.ncbi.nlm.nih.gov/pubmed/24680621, (2019 October 11).

[26] Hannan A., Saleem S., Chaudhary S., Barkaat M., Arshad MU, "Anti bacterial activity of Nigella sativa against clinical isolates of methicillin resistant Staphylococcus aureus," https://www.ncbi.nlm.nih.gov, https://www.ncbi.nlm.nih.gov/pubmed/19610522, (2019 October 11)

[27] Dehkordi FR, Kamkhah AF, "Antihypertensive effect of Nigella sativa seed extract in patients with mild hypertension," https://www.ncbi.

nlm.nih.gov. https://www.ncbi.nlm.nih.gov/pubmed/18705755, (2019 October 11)

[28] Jing Yang,[1] Jinhua Yin,[1,2] Hongfei Gao,[1] Linxin Xu,[1,2] Yan Wang,[1] Lu Xu,[2] and Ming Li[2] "Berberine Improves Insulin Sensitivity by Inhibiting Fat Store and Adjusting Adipokines Profile in Human Preadipocytes and Metabolic Syndrome Patients," www.hindawi.com, https://www.hindawi.com/journals/ecam/2012/363845/, (2019 March 2)

[29] Vasilios G. Athyros, "The use of statins alone, or in combination with pioglitazone and other drugs, for the treatment of non-alcoholic fatty liver disease/non-alcoholic steatohepatitis and related cardiovascular risk," https://www.metabolismjournal.com/article/S0026-0495(17)30075-6/fulltext. (2019 March 1).

[30] Jeffery, Elizabeth, "Myrosinase," https://www.sciencedirect.com, https://www.sciencedirect.com/topics/biochemistry-genetics-and-molecular-biology/myrosinase, (2019 August 10)

[31] Zhao Jing, Moore Anthony N., Clifton Guy L., Dash Pramod K, "Sulforaphane enhances aquaporin–4 expression and decreases cerebral edema following traumatic brain injury," https://onlinelibrary.wiley.com. https://onlinelibrary.wiley.com/doi/full/10.1002/jnr.20649, (2019 August 24)

[32] Egner, Patricia, "Rapid and Sustainable Detoxication of Airborne Pollutants by Broccoli Sprout Beverage: Results of a Randomized Clinical Trial in China," https://cancerpreventionresearch.aacrjournals.org, https://cancerpreventionresearch.aacrjournals.org/content/early/2014/06/07/1940-6207.CAPR-14-0103, (2019 August 22)

[33] Ritz Stacey, Wan Junxiang, Diaz-Sanchez David, "Sulforaphane-stimulated phase II enzyme induction inhibits cytokine production by airway epithelial cells stimulated with diesel extract," https://www.physiology.org, https://www.physiology.org/doi/full/10.1152/ajplung.00170.2006, (2019 August 22)

[34] Chang YW, Jang JY, Kim YH, Kim JW, Shim JJ, "The Effects of Broccoli Sprout Extract Containing Sulforaphane on Lipid Peroxidation and Helicobacter pylori Infection in the Gastric Mucosa," https://www.ncbi.nlm.nih.gov, https://www.ncbi.nlm.nih.gov/pubmed/25287166, (2019 August 21)

35   Fahey JW, Stephenson KK, Wade KL, Talalay P., "Urease from Helicobacter pylori is inactivated by sulforaphane and other isothiocyanates," https://www.ncbi.nlm.nih.gov, https://www.ncbi.nlm.nih.gov/pubmed/23583386, (2019 August 21)

36   Tortorella SM, Royce SG, Licciardi PV, Karagiannis TC, "Dietary Sulforaphane in Cancer Chemoprevention: The Role of Epigenetic Regulation and HDAC Inhibition," https://www.ncbi.nlm.nih.gov, https://www.ncbi.nlm.nih.gov/pmc/articles/PMC4432495/, (2019 August 21)

37   Ho GT, Wangensteen H, Barsett H., "Elderberry and Elderflower Extracts, Phenolic Compounds, and Metabolites and Their Effect on Complement, RAW 264.7 Macrophages and Dendritic Cells," https://www.ncbi.nlm.nih.gov, https://www.ncbi.nlm.nih.gov/pmc/articles/PMC5372600/, (2019 March 5)

38   Lila MA, "Anthocyanins and Human Health: An In Vitro Investigative Approach," https://www.ncbi.nlm.nih.gov, https://www.ncbi.nlm.nih.gov/pmc/articles/PMC1082894/, (2019 March 5)

39   Farrell N, Norris G, Lee SG, Chun OK, Blesso CN, "Anthocyanin-rich black elderberry extract improves markers of HDL function and reduces aortic cholesterol in hyperlipidemic mice," https://www.ncbi.nlm.nih.gov, https://www.ncbi.nlm.nih.gov/pubmed/25758596, (2019 March 5)

40   Zakay-Rones Z, Thom E, Wollan T, Wadstein J., "Randomized study of the efficacy and safety of oral elderberry extract in the treatment of influenza A and B virus infections," https://www.ncbi.nlm.nih.gov, https://www.ncbi.nlm.nih.gov/pubmed/15080016, (2019 March 5)

41   Tiralongo E, Wee SS, Lea RA," Elderberry Supplementation Reduces Cold Duration and Symptoms in Air-Travellers: A Randomized, Double-Blind Placebo-Controlled Clinical Trial," https://www.ncbi.nlm.nih.gov, https://www.ncbi.nlm.nih.gov/pmc/articles/PMC4848651/, (2019 March 5)

42   Melzer J, Saller R, Schapowal A, Brignoli R., "Systematic review of clinical data with BNO-101 (Sinupret) in the treatment of sinusitis," https://www.ncbi.nlm.nih.gov, https://www.ncbi.nlm.nih.gov/pubmed/16645287, (2019 March 5)

43 Thole JM, Kraft TF, Sueiro LA, Kang YH, Gills JJ, Cuendet M, Pezzuto JM, Seigler DS, Lila MA," A comparative evaluation of the anticancer properties of European and American elderberry fruits," https://www.ncbi.nlm.nih.gov, https://www.ncbi.nlm.nih.gov/pubmed/17201636, (2019 March 5)

44 Gray AM, Abdel-Wahab YH, Flatt PR, "The traditional plant treatment, Sambucus nigra (elder), exhibits insulin-like and insulin-releasing actions in vitro," https://www.ncbi.nlm.nih.gov, https://www.ncbi.nlm.nih.gov/pubmed/10613759, (2019 March 5)

45 Wright CI, Van-Buren L, Kroner CI, Koning MM, "Herbal medicines as diuretics: a review of the scientific evidence," https://www.ncbi.nlm.nih.gov, https://www.ncbi.nlm.nih.gov/pubmed/17804183, (2019 March 5)

46 Feskanich D, Ziegler RG, Michaud DS, Giovannucci EL, Speizer FE, Willett WC, Colditz GA, "Prospective study of fruit and vegetable consumption and risk of lung cancer among men and women," https://www.ncbi.nlm.nih.gov, https://www.ncbi.nlm.nih.gov/pubmed/11078758, (2018 April 3)

47 Larson RD, Holly, "The Beginner's Guide to Cruciferous Vegetables," https://www.eatright.org, https://www.eatright.org/food/vitamins-and-supplements/nutrient-rich-foods/the-beginners-guide-to-cruciferous-vegetables, (2018 April 14)

48 National Cancer Institute, "Cruciferous Vegetables and Cancer Prevention" https://www.cancer.gov, https://www.cancer.gov/about-cancer/causes-prevention/risk/diet/cruciferous-vegetables-factsheet?redirect=true, (2019 May 3)

49 Murillo G, Mehta RG, "Cruciferous vegetables and cancer prevention," https://www.ncbi.nlm.nih.gov, https://www.ncbi.nlm.nih.gov/pubmed/12094621, (2018 April 3)

50 Mehta RG, Liu J, Constantinou A, Thomas CF, Hawthorne M, You M, Gerhüser C, Pezzuto JM, Moon RC, Moriarty RM, "Cancer chemopreventive activity of brassinin, a phytoalexin from cabbage," https://www.ncbi.nlm.nih.gov, https://www.ncbi.nlm.nih.gov/pubmed/7859373, (2018 March 26)

51 Weber P., "Vitamin K and bone health," https://www.ncbi.nlm.nih.gov, https://www.ncbi.nlm.nih.gov/pubmed/11684396, (2018 April 8)

52 LLC, Webmd, "Folic Acid," https://www.webmd.com, https://www.webmd.com/baby/folic-acid-and-pregnancy#1, (2018 April 8)

53 He FJ, MacGregor GA, "Beneficial effects of potassium on human health," https://www.ncbi.nlm.nih.gov, https://www.ncbi.nlm.nih.gov/pubmed/18724413, (2018 March 7)

54 Jegtvig, Shereen, "Can a healthy diet prevent cataracts?" https://www.allaboutvision.com, https://www.allaboutvision.com/nutrition/cataracts.htm, (2018 April 9)

55 Price, Annie, "Brazil Nuts," www.draxe.com, https://draxe.com/nutrition/brazil-nuts/, (2018 February 11)

56 "Coffee and Your Health," Osterweil, Neil, https://www.webmd.com, https://www.webmd.com/food-recipes/features/coffee-new-health-food#1, (2019 March 4)

57 RD Link, Rachel, "Is Coffee Good or Bad for You? Coffee Nutrition Facts vs Fiction," www.draxe.com, https://draxe.com/nutrition/coffee-nutrition-facts/, (2018 February 12)

58 McLaren DS, "Vitamin A Deficiency Disorders," https://www.ncbi.nlm.nih.gov, https://www.ncbi.nlm.nih.gov/pubmed/10643184, (2019 June 4)

59 Nurk E, Refsum H, Drevon CA, Tell GS, Nygaard HA, Engedal K, Smith AD, "Cognitive performance among the elderly in relation to the intake of plant foods, The Hordaland Health Study," https://www.ncbi.nlm.nih.gov, https://www.ncbi.nlm.nih.gov/pubmed/20550741, (2019 May 28)

60 Ramesh Kandimalla, P. Hemachandra Reddy, "Therapeutics of Neurotransmitters in Alzheimer's Disease," https://www.ncbi.nlm.nih.gov, https://www.ncbi.nlm.nih.gov/pmc/articles/PMC5793221/, (2019 May 5)

61 Ruggeri, Christine, "Chia seeds vs flax seeds: Which is Healthier?" www.draxe.com, https://draxe.com/nutrition/chia-seeds-vs-flax-seeds/, (2018 February 21)

62 Bae JM, Kim EH, "Dietary intakes of citrus fruit and risk of gastric cancer incidence: an adaptive meta-analysis of cohort studies," https://www.ncbi.nlm.nih.gov, https://www.ncbi.nlm.nih.gov/pmc/articles/PMC5037356/, (2018 March 17)

63   Price, Annie, "Cantaloupe Nutrition: The Phytonutrient Powerhouse You May Be Overlooking," www.draxe.com, https://draxe.com/nutrition/cantaloupe-nutrition/, (2018 March 14)

64   Christensen LP, Brandt K., "Bioactive polyacetylenes in food plants of the Apiaceae family: occurrence, bioactivity and analysis," https://www.ncbi.nlm.nih.gov, https://www.ncbi.nlm.nih.gov/pubmed/16520011,_(2018 October 28)

65   RD Olsen, Natalie, "Does celery juice have health benefits?" www.medicalnewstoday.com, https://www.medicalnewstoday.com/articles/324932.php, (2019 June 2)

66   Ruggeri, Christine, "Benefits of Cherries: Weight Loss, Gout Healing & Less Inflammation!" www.draxe.com, https://draxe.com/nutrition/benefits-of-cherries/, (2018 April 19)

67   Pham-Huy LA, He H, Pham-Huy C., "Free radicals, antioxidants in disease and health," https://www.ncbi.nlm.nih.gov, https://www.ncbi.nlm.nih.gov/pmc/articles/PMC3614697/, (2019 January 23)

68   LLC, Webmd, "Cats-Claw," https://www.webmd.com, https://www.webmd.com/vitamins/ai/ingredientmono-395/cats-claw, (2018 November 1)

69   Riva L, Coradini D, Di Fronzo G, De Feo V, De Tommasi N, De Simone F, Pizza C., "The antiproliferative effects of Uncaria tomentosa extracts and fractions on the growth of breast cancer cell line," https://www.ncbi.nlm.nih.gov, https://www.ncbi.nlm.nih.gov/pubmed/11724307, (2019 March 17)

70   Price, Annie, "8 Cat's Claw Benefits for Immunity, Digestion & Chronic Disease," www.draxe.com, https://draxe.com/nutrition/cats-claw/, (2018 April 23)

71   RD Grieger, Lynn, "VITAMIN K AND BONE HEALTH," https://www.summitmedicalgroup.com, https://www.summitmedicalgroup.com/news/nutrition/vitamin-k-and-bone-health/, (2019 May 23)

72   Nishimura M, Ohkawara T, Kanayama T, Kitagawa K, Nishimura H, Nishihira J., "Effects of the extract from roasted chicory (Cichorium intybus L.) root containing inulin-type fructans on blood glucose, lipid metabolism, and fecal properties," www.ncbi.nlm.nih.gov, https://www.ncbi.nlm.nih.gov/pubmed/26151029, (2019 June 4)

[73] Levy, Jillian, "Cashews Nutrition: Helps Prevent Cancer, Diabetes & More," www.draxe.com, https://draxe.com/nutrition/cashews-nutrition/, (2018 May 1)

[74] Dr. Axe, Josh, "7 Proven Chlorella Benefits (#2 is Best)," www.draxe.com. https://draxe.com/nutrition/7-proven-chlorella-benefits-side-effects/, (2018 May 3)

[75] LLC, Webmd, "Chlorella," www.wedmd.com, https://www.webmd.com/vitamins-and-supplements/chlorella-uses-and-risks, (2018 May 15)

[76] Villines, Zawn,"What you need to know about tocotrienols," https://www.medicalnewstoday.com, https://www.medicalnewstoday.com/articles/319689.php, (2019 May 13)

[77] Pullar JM, Carr AC, Vissers MCM, "The Roles of Vitamin C in Skin Health," https://www.ncbi.nlm.nih.gov, https://www.ncbi.nlm.nih.gov/pubmed/28805671, (2018 September 30)

[78] RD Link, Rachael, "Dragon Fruit Benefits, Including for Anti-Aging and Heart Health," www.draxe.com, https://draxe.com/nutrition/dragon-fruit-benefits/, (2018 May 5)

[79] Holzapfel NP, Shokoohmand A, Wagner F, Landgraf M, Champ S, Holzapfel BM, Clements JA, Hutmacher DW, Loessner D., "Lycopene reduces ovarian tumor growth and intraperitoneal metastatic load," https://www.ncbi.nlm.nih.gov, https://www.ncbi.nlm.nih.gov/pubmed/28670494, (2019 June 5)

[80] Oliver, Kyra, "8 Surprising Dill Weed Benefits (#6 Is Energizing)," www.draxe.com, https://draxe.com/nutrition/dill-weed/, (2018 May 17)

[81] Nurk E, Refsum H, Drevon CA, Tell GS, Nygaard HA, Engedal K, Smith AD, "Intake of flavonoid-rich wine, tea, and chocolate by elderly men and women is associated with better cognitive test performance," https://www.ncbi.nlm.nih.gov, https://www.ncbi.nlm.nih.gov/pubmed/19056649, (2018 May 24)

[82] Levy, Jillian, "7 Eggplant Health Benefits and Nutritional Information," www.draxe.com, https://draxe.com/nutrition/eggplant-nutrition/, (2018 May 30)

[83] Levy, Jillian, "7 Eggplant Health Benefits and Nutritional Information," www.draxe.com, https://draxe.com/nutrition/eggplant-nutrition/, (2018 May 30)

84 Oliver, Kyra, "Slippery Elm: The Digestive Aid that May Fight Breast Cancer," www.draxe.com, https://draxe.com/nutrition/slippery-elm/, (2018 June 2)

85 Group, Dr. Edward, "What are Carotenoids?- 5 Health Benefits," https://www.globalhealingcenter.com, https://www.globalhealingcenter.com/natural-health/what-are-carotenoids/, (2018 November 20)

86 Gilbert, Monique, "The Healing Power of Soy's Isoflavones," https://www.fwhc.org, https://www.fwhc.org/health/soy.htm, (2018 November 23)

87 Ruggeri, Christine, "Fennel Benefits, Nutrition & Fantastic Recipes," www.draxe.com, https://draxe.com/nutrition/fennel-benefits/, (2019 January 12)

88 Dohadwala MM, Vita JA, "Grapes and cardiovascular disease," https://www.ncbi.nlm.nih.gov, https://www.ncbi.nlm.nih.gov/pubmed/19625699, (2019 February 14)

89 Okudan, Nilsel; Belviranli, Muaz,"Well-Known Antioxidants and Newcomers in Sport Nutrition Coenzyme Q10, Quercetin, Resveratrol, Pterostilbene, Pycnogenol and Astaxanthin" https://www.ncbi.nlm.nih.gov.https://www.ncbi.nlm.nih.gov/books/NBK299046/, (2019 October 10)

90 Dr. Axe, Josh, "How Grapes Nutrition Boost Health, Including Your Brain," www.draxe.com, https://draxe.com/nutrition/grapes-nutrition/, (2019 February 14)

91 Bae JM, Lee EJ, Guyatt G., "Citrus fruit intake and pancreatic cancer risk: a quantitative systematic review," https://www.ncbi.nlm.nih.gov, https://www.ncbi.nlm.nih.gov/pubmed/18824947, (2018 March 19)

92 RD Link, Rachael, "Guava: Powerful Antioxidant Food for Your Immune System," www.draxe.com, https://draxe.com/nutrition/guava/, (2019 May 10)

93 YangGaoMin-feiYangYa-pingSuHui-minJiangXiao-juanYouYin-jingYangHai-longZhang, "Ginsenoside Re reduces insulin resistance through activation of PPAR-γ pathway and inhibition of TNF-α production," https://www.sciencedirect.com, https://www.sciencedirect.com/science/article/pii/S0378874113002134?via%3Dihub, (2018 December 10)

94   Murphy LL, Lee TJ, "Ginseng, sex behavior, and nitric oxide," https://www.ncbi.nlm.nih.gov.   https://www.ncbi.nlm.nih.gov/pubmed/12076988, (2018 December 11)

95   Semwal RB, Semwal DK, Combrinck S, Viljoen AM, "Gingerols and shogaols: Important nutraceutical principles from ginger," https://www.ncbi.nlm.nih.gov, https://www.ncbi.nlm.nih.gov/pubmed/26228533, (2018 December 12)

96   Hill, Ansley, "12 Benefits of Gingko Biloba (Plus side effects and Dosage)," https://www.healthline.com, https://www.healthline.com/nutrition/ginkgo-biloba-benefits#section1, (2019 April 6)

97   RD Link, Rachael, "10 Proven Manuka Honey Benefits and Uses," www.draxe.com, https://draxe.com/nutrition/manuka-honey-benefits-uses/, (2019 March 2)

98   Yin G, Cao L, Xu P, Jeney G, Nakao M., "Hepatoprotective and antioxidant effects of Hibiscus sabdariffa extract against carbon tetrachloride-induced hepatocyte damage in Cyprinus carpio," https://www.ncbi.nlm.nih.gov, https://www.ncbi.nlm.nih.gov/pubmed/21082285, (2019 July 14)

99   Chang HC, Peng CH, Yeh DM, Kao ES, Wang CJ, "Hibiscus sabdariffa extract inhibits obesity and fat accumulation, and improves liver steatosis in humans," https://www.ncbi.nlm.nih.gov, https://www.ncbi.nlm.nih.gov/pubmed/24549255, (2018 August 11)

100   Edwards, Rebekah, "Hibiscus Tea: The Antioxidant 'Therapeutic Agent' You Should Be Drinking," www.draxe.com, https://draxe.com/nutrition/hibiscus-tea/, (2019 March 15)

101   Campbell, Damien, "Interesting Facts About the Hackberry Tree," https://www.sciencing.com, https://sciencing.com/interesting-hackberry-tree-6513384.html, (2019 June 16)

102   Ruggeri, Christine, "Hemp Seeds Benefits for Pain, Weight Loss and More," www.draxe.com, https://draxe.com/nutrition/7-hemp-seed-benefits-nutrition-profile/, (2019 May 2)

103   LLC, Webmd, "Gamma Linolenic Acid," https://www.webmd.com, https://www.webmd.com/vitamins/ai/ingredientmono-805/gamma-linolenic-acid, (2019 June 13)

[104] Slavin J."Fiber and prebiotics: mechanisms and health benefits," https://www.ncbi.nlm.nih.gov, https://www.ncbi.nlm.nih.gov/pmc/articles/PMC3705355/, (2019 July 6)

[105] American Diabetes Association, "Fruit," https://www.diabetes.org, https://www.diabetes.org/nutrition/healthy-food-choices-made-easy/fruit, (2019 March 30)

[106] Sunita P, Pattanayak SP, "Phytoestrogens in postmenopausal indications: A theoretical perspective," https://www.ncbi.nlm.nih.gov, https://www.ncbi.nlm.nih.gov/pmc/articles/PMC3210008/, (2019 July 27)

[107] Levy, Jillian, "11 Juniper Berry Essential Oil Uses + Benefits," www.draxe.com, https://draxe.com/essential-oils/juniper-berry-essential-oil/, (2019 October 5)

[108] de Oliveira Leite AM, Miguel MA, Peixoto RS, Rosado AS, Silva JT, Paschoalin VM, "Microbiological, technological and therapeutic properties of kefir: a natural probiotic beverage," https://www.ncbi.nlm.nih.gov, https://www.ncbi.nlm.nih.gov/pmc/articles/PMC3833126/, (2018 December 19)

[109] Van Duyn MA, Pivonka E., "Overview of the health benefits of fruit and vegetable consumption for the dietetics professional: selected literature," https://www.ncbi.nlm.nih.gov, https://www.ncbi.nlm.nih.gov/pubmed/11138444, (2019 August 13)

[110] National Cancer Institute, "Cruciferous Vegetables and Cancer Prevention," https://www.cancer.gov, https://www.cancer.gov/about-cancer/causes-prevention/risk/diet/cruciferous-vegetables-fact-sheet?redirect=true, (2019 May 3)

[111] Lee CJ, Wilson L, Jordan MA, Nguyen V, Tang J, Smiyun G., "Hesperidin suppressed proliferations of both human breast cancer and androgen-dependent prostate cancer cells," https://www.ncbi.nlm.nih.gov, https://www.ncbi.nlm.nih.gov/pubmed/19548283, (2019 February 11)

[112] Crowell PL, Gould MN, "Chemoprevention and therapy of cancer by d-limonene," https://www.ncbi.nlm.nih.gov, https://www.ncbi.nlm.nih.gov/pubmed/7948106, (2019 April 6)

[113] Staughton, John, "10 Best Benefits of Loquat," https://www.organicfacts.net, https://www.organicfacts.net/health-benefits/fruit/loquat.html, (2019 July 12)

114   Mercola, Dr. Joseph, "What is Longan Good For?" https://www. foodfacts.mercola.com, https://foodfacts.mercola.com/longan.html, (2019 July 13)

115   O'Brien, Sharon, "4 Impressive Health Benefits of Lysine," https://www. healthline.com, https://www.healthline.com/nutrition/lysine-benefits, (2018 December 12)

116   Mozaffarieh M, Sacu S, Wedrich A, "The role of the carotenoids, lutein and zeaxanthin, in protecting against age-related macular degeneration: a review based on controversial evidence," https://www.ncbi.nlm.nih. gov, https://www.ncbi.nlm.nih.gov/pmc/articles/PMC305368/, (2019 January 22)

117   Adukwu EC, Allen SC, Phillips CA, "The anti-biofilm activity of lemongrass (Cymbopogon flexuosus) and grapefruit (Citrus paradisi) essential oils against five strains of Staphylococcus aureus," https://www. ncbi.nlm.nih.gov, https://www.ncbi.nlm.nih.gov/pubmed/22862808, (2019 March 8)

118   Okigbo RN, Mmeka EC, "Antimicrobial effects of three tropical plant extracts on Staphylococcus aureus, Escherichia coli and Candida albicans," https://www.ncbi.nlm.nih.gov, https://www.ncbi.nlm.nih.gov/ pmc/articles/PMC2816559/, (2019 April 17)

119   Aiemsaard J, Aiumlamai S, Aromdee C, Taweechaisupapong S, Khunkitti W., "The effect of lemongrass oil and its major components on clinical isolate mastitis pathogens and their mechanisms of action on Staphylococcus aureus DMST 4745," https://www.ncbi.nlm.nih.gov, https://www.ncbi.nlm.nih.gov/pubmed/21316719, (2019 March 8)

120   Cavanagh HM, Wilkinson JM, "Biological activities of lavender essential oil," https://www.ncbi.nlm.nih.gov, https://www.ncbi.nlm.nih.gov/ pubmed/12112282/, (2019 January 13)

121   Tabassum N, Hamdani M., "Plants used to treat skin diseases," https:// www.ncbi.nlm.nih.gov, https://www.ncbi.nlm.nih.gov/pmc/articles/ PMC3931201/, (2019 January 9)

122   de Rapper S, Kamatou G, Viljoen A, van Vuuren S., "The In Vitro Antimicrobial Activity of Lavandula angustifolia Essential Oil in Combination with Other Aroma-Therapeutic Oils," https://www.ncbi.

nlm.nih.gov, https://www.ncbi.nlm.nih.gov/pubmed/23737850, (2019 January 12)

123 Sebai H, Selmi S, Rtibi K, Souli A, Gharbi N, Sakly M., "Lavender (Lavandula stoechas L.) essential oils attenuate hyperglycemia and protect against oxidative stress in alloxan-induced diabetic rats," https://www.ncbi.nlm.nih.gov, https://www.ncbi.nlm.nih.gov/pmc/articles/PMC3880178/, (2019 January 12)

124 Mori HM, Kawanami H, Kawahata H, Aoki M., "Wound healing potential of lavender oil by acceleration of granulation and wound contraction through induction of TGF-β in a rat model," https://www.ncbi.nlm.nih.gov, https://www.ncbi.nlm.nih.gov/pmc/articles/PMC4880962/, (2019 January 11)

125 Xu P, Wang K, Lu C, Dong L, Gao L, Yan M, Aibai S, Yang Y, Liu X., "The Protective Effect of Lavender Essential Oil and Its Main Component Linalool against the Cognitive Deficits Induced by D-Galactose and Aluminum Trichloride in Mice," https://www.ncbi.nlm.nih.gov, https://www.ncbi.nlm.nih.gov/pmc/articles/PMC5424179/, (2019 January 5)

126 Hancianu M, Cioanca O, Mihasan M, Hritcu L., "Neuroprotective effects of inhaled lavender oil on scopolamine-induced dementia via anti-oxidative activities in rats," https://www.ncbi.nlm.nih.gov, https://www.ncbi.nlm.nih.gov/pubmed/23351960, (2019 January 7)

127 Sasannejad P., Saeedi M., Shoeibi A., Gorji A., Abbasi M., Foroughipour M., "Lavender essential oil in the treatment of migraine headache: a placebo-controlled clinical trial," https://www.ncbi.nlm.nih.gov, https://www.ncbi.nlm.nih.gov/pubmed/22517298, (2019 January 2)

128 Hirokawa K, Nishimoto T, Taniguchi T., "Effects of lavender aroma on sleep quality in healthy Japanese students," https://www.ncbi.nlm.nih.gov, https://www.ncbi.nlm.nih.gov/pmc/articles/PMC3612440/#B74, (2019 January 2)

129 Keshavarz Afshar M, Behboodi Moghadam Z, Taghizadeh Z, Bekhradi R, Montazeri A, Mokhtari P., "Lavender fragrance essential oil and the quality of sleep in postpartum women," https://www.ncbi.nlm.nih.gov, https://www.ncbi.nlm.nih.gov/pmc/articles/PMC4443384/, (2019 January 2)

[130] Conrad P, Adams C., "The effects of clinical aromatherapy for anxiety and depression in the high-risk postpartum woman - a pilot study," https://www.ncbi.nlm.nih.gov, https://www.ncbi.nlm.nih.gov/pubmed/22789792, (2019 January 2)

[131] Ivanova D, Gerova D, Chervenkov T, Yankova T., Polyphenols and antioxidant capacity of Bulgarian medicinal plants. J Ethnopharmacol, 2005 Jan 4; 96(1-2):145-50

[132] Brantner A, Kartnig T., "Flavonoid glycosides from aerial parts of Pulmonaria officinalis," Planta Med, 1995 Dec; 61(6):582, https://www.ncbi.nlm.nih.gov/pmc/articles/PMC4329619/, (2019 July 12).

[133] Group, Dr., "A Brief History of Lungwort," https://www.alrightnow.com. https://www.alrightnow.com/the-lung-cleansing-benefits-of-lungwort/, (2019 May 29).

[134] Liu LK, Lee HJ, Shih YW, Chyau CC, Wang CJ, "Mulberry anthocyanin extracts inhibit LDL oxidation and macrophage-derived foam cell formation induced by oxidative LDL," https://www.ncbi.nlm.nih.gov, https://www.ncbi.nlm.nih.gov/pubmed/19241587, (2019 July 15)

[135] Chang JJ, Hsu MJ, Huang HP, Chung DJ, Chang YC, Wang CJ, "Mulberry anthocyanins inhibit oleic acid induced lipid accumulation by reduction of lipogenesis and promotion of hepatic lipid clearance," https://www.ncbi.nlm.nih.gov, https://www.ncbi.nlm.nih.gov/pubmed/23731091, (2019 July 15)

[136] Abenavoli L, Capasso R, Milic N, Capasso F., "Milk thistle in liver diseases: past, present, future," https://www.ncbi.nlm.nih.gov, https://www.ncbi.nlm.nih.gov/pubmed/20564545, (2019 March 18)

[137] Katiyar SK, Meleth S, Sharma SD, "Silymarin, a flavonoid from milk thistle (Silybum marianum L.), inhibits UV-induced oxidative stress through targeting infiltrating CD11b+ cells in mouse skin," https://www.ncbi.nlm.nih.gov, https://www.ncbi.nlm.nih.gov/pmc/articles/PMC2394725/, (2019 March 18)

[138] LLC, WebMD, "Manganese," https://www.webmd.com, https://www.webmd.com/vitamins/ai/ingredientmono-182/manganese, (2018 October 23)

[139] PH.D Higdon, Jane, " Manganese," https://lpi.oregostate.edu, https://lpi.oregonstate.edu/mic/minerals/manganese, (2019 August 15)

140   Cloyd, Raymond, "Explaining Azadirachtin and Neem," https://gpnmag.com, https://gpnmag.com/article/explaining-azadirachtin-and-neem/, (2019 January 15)

141   Ann Thomas, Rancy; Krishnakumari, Dr., "Lipid Lowering Effects of Myristica Fragrans," https://semanticscholar.org, https://pdfs.semanticscholar.org/b5b0/6771a9aba3d66b171f8062cc72198732a65f.pdf, (2019 June 15)

142   Mozaffarieh M, Sacu S, Wedrich A., "The role of the carotenoids, lutein and zeaxanthin, in protecting against age-related macular degeneration: a review based on controversial evidence," https://www.ncbi.nlm.nih.gov, https://www.ncbi.nlm.nih.gov/pmc/articles/PMC305368/, (2019 January 22)

143   Susalit E, Agus N, Effendi I, Tjandrawinata RR, Nofiarny D, Perrinjaquet-Moccetti T, Verbruggen M., "Olive (Olea europaea) leaf extract effective in patients with stage-1 hypertension: comparison with Captopril," https://www.ncbi.nlm.nih.gov. https://www.ncbi.nlm.nih.gov/pubmed/21036583, (2019 September 7)

144   Ruggeri, Christine, "Olive Leaf Extract Benefits for Cardiovascular Health and Brain Function," www.draxe.com, https://draxe.com/nutrition/olive-leaf-benefits/, (2019 September 3)

145   Kontogianni VG, Charisiadis P, Margianni E, Lamari FN, Gerothanassis IP, Tzakos AG, "Olive leaf extracts are a natural source of advanced glycation end product inhibitors," https://www.ncbi.nlm.nih.gov, https://www.ncbi.nlm.nih.gov/pubmed/24044491, (2019 August 10)

146   Joshipura KJ, Hu FB, Manson JE, Stampfer MJ, Rimm EB, Speizer FE, Colditz G, Ascherio A, Rosner B, Spiegelman D, Willett WC, "The effect of fruit and vegetable intake on risk for coronary heart disease," https://www.ncbi.nlm.nih.gov, https://www.ncbi.nlm.nih.gov/pubmed/11412050, (2019 January 3)

147   Yamada T, Hayasaka S, Shibata Y, Ojima T, Saegusa T, Gotoh T, Ishikawa S, Nakamura Y, Kayaba K., "Frequency of citrus fruit intake is associated with the incidence of cardiovascular disease: the Jichi Medical School cohort study," https://www.ncbi.nlm.nih.gov, https://www.ncbi.nlm.nih.gov/pmc/articles/PMC3899405/, (2018 January 13)

148   Othman RA, Moghadasian MH, Jones PJ, "Cholesterol-lowering effects of oat β-glucan," https://www.ncbi.nlm.nih.gov, https://www.ncbi.nlm.nih.gov/pubmed/21631511, (2018 November 18)

149   Griffiths G, Trueman L, Crowther T, Thomas B, Smith B., "Onions—a global benefit to health," https://www.ncbi.nlm.nih.gov, https://www.ncbi.nlm.nih.gov/pubmed/12410539, (2019 June 7)

150   Khaki A, Fathiazad F, Nouri M, Khaki AA, Khamenehi HJ, Hamadeh M., "Evaluation of androgenic activity of allium cepa on spermatogenesis in the rat," https:www.ncbi.nlm.nih.gov, https://www.ncbi.nlm.nih.gov/pubmed/19384830, (2018 October 11)

151   RDN Kaufman, Caroline, "Foods That Can affect Fertility," https://www.eatright.org, https://www.eatright.org/health/pregnancy/fertility-and-reproduction/fertility-foods, (2019 March 23)

152   Group, Dr. Edward, "What Is Carvacrol? 8 Facts to Know," https://www.globalhealingcenter.com, https://www.globalhealingcenter.com/natural-health/what-is-carvacrol-8-facts-to-know/, (2019 September 8)

153   Costa-Orlandi CB, Sardi JCO, Pitangui NS, de Oliveira HC, Scorzoni L, Galeane MC, Medina-Alarcón KP, Melo WCMA, Marcelino MY, Braz JD, Fusco-Almeida AM, Mendes-Giannini MJS, "Fungal Biofilms and Polymicrobial Diseases," https://www.ncbi.nlm.nih.gov, https://www.ncbi.nlm.nih.gov/pmc/articles/PMC5715925/, (2019 July 5)

154   LLC, Webmd, " Bromelain" https://www.webmd.com, https://www.webmd.com/vitamins/ai/ingredientmono-895/bromelain, (2018 February 9)

155   LLC, Webmd, "Tryptophan," https://www.webmd.com, https://www.webmd.com/vitamins/ai/ingredientmono-326/l-tryptophan, (2019 July 2)

156   Mcdermott, Annette, "6 Ways to use Papain" https://www.healthline.com, https://www.healthline.com/health/food-nutrition/papain, (2019 September 18)

157   Sathasivam K, Ramanathan S, Mansor SM, Haris MR, Wernsdorfer WH, "Thrombocyte counts in mice after the administration of papaya leaf suspension," https://www.ncbi.nlm.nih.gov/pubmed/19915811, https://www.ncbi.nlm.nih.gov, (2019 September 28)

158 Fischier Rachel, Ben-Amotz, Ami, "Analysis of carotenoids with emphasis on 9-*cis* β-carotene in vegetables and fruits commonly consumed in Israel," https://www.sciencedirect.com, https://www.sciencedirect.com/science/article/pii/S0308814697001969, (2019 April 2)

159 DO Cunha, John, "Boron," https://www.rxlist.com. https://www.rxlist.com/consumer_boron/drugs-condition.htm, (2018 January 20)

160 Zhang J, Ping W, Chunrong W, Shou CX, Keyou G., "Nonhypercholesterolemic effects of a palm oil diet in Chinese adults," https://www.ncbi.nlm.nih.gov, https://www.ncbi.nlm.nih.gov/pubmed/9082037, (2019 June 23)

161 R.D. Zeratsky, Katherine, "I've seen prickly pear cactus promoted as a superfood. What's behind the hype?" https://www.mayoclinic.org, https://www.mayoclinic.org/healthy-lifestyle/consumer-health/expert-answers/prickly-pear-cactus/faq-20057771, (2019 August 15)

162 McKay DL, "A review of the bioactivity and potential health benefits of peppermint tea (Mentha piperita L.)," https://www.ncbi.nlm.nih.gov, https://www.ncbi.nlm.nih.gov/m/pubmed/16767798/, (2019 February 12)

163 Meamarbashi A., "Instant effects of peppermint essential oil on the physiological parameters and exercise performance," https://www.ncbi.nlm.nih.gov, https://www.ncbi.nlm.nih.gov/pmc/articles/PMC4103722/, (2019 February 12)

164 Benjamin Kligler, Sapna Chaudhary, "Peppermint Oil," https://www.semanticscholar.org, https://www.semanticscholar.org/paper/Peppermint-oil-Kligler-Chaudhary/67caf71840bc726676755c8531f6c6bd9fa576cc, (2019 February 1)

165 Orchard A, van Vuuren S., "Commercial Essential Oils as Potential Antimicrobials to Treat Skin Diseases," https://www.ncbi.nlm.nih.gov, https://www.ncbi.nlm.nih.gov/pmc/articles/PMC5435909/, (2019 March 1)

166 Oh JY, Park MA, Kim YC, "Peppermint Oil Promotes Hair Growth without Toxic Signs," https://www.ncbi.nlm.nih.gov, https://www.ncbi.nlm.nih.gov/pmc/articles/PMC4289931/, (2019 February 9)

167 Alves JG, de Brito Rde C, Cavalcanti TS, "Effectiveness of Mentha piperita in the Treatment of Infantile Colic: A Crossover Study," https://

www.ncbi.nlm.nih.gov, https://www.ncbi.nlm.nih.gov/pmc/articles/ PMC3403674/, (2019 February 13)

168 Thosar N, Basak S, Bahadure RN, Rajurkar M., "Antimicrobial efficacy of five essential oils against oral pathogens: An in vitro study," https:// www.ncbi.nlm.nih.gov, https://www.ncbi.nlm.nih.gov/pmc/articles/ PMC4054083/, (2019 February 12)

169 Reporter, The Daily Mail, "Viagara Effect from a daily glass of pomegranate juice," https://www.dailymail.co.uk/sciencetech/ article-2139292/Viagra-effect-daily-glass-pomegranate-juice.html, (2019 April 16)

170 Grossman, Michael E., "Punicic acid is an omega-5 fatty acid capable of inhibiting breast cancer proliferation," https://www.semanticscholar.org. https://www.semanticscholar.org/paper/Punicic-acid-is-an-omega-5-fatty-acid-capable-of-Grossmann-Mizuno/63843b0589524d16919441de68bb1343b09b70cf, (2019 August 3)

171 Asgary S, Keshvari M, Sahebkar A, Hashemi M, Rafieian-Kopaei M., "Clinical investigation of the acute effects of pomegranate juice on blood pressure and endothelial function in hypertensive individuals," https://www.ncbi.nlm.nih.gov, https://www.ncbi.nlm.nih.gov/ pubmed/24575134, (2019 September 21)

172 Grether-Beck S, Marini A, Jaenicke T, Krutmann J., "French Maritime Pine Bark Extract (Pycnogenol®) Effects on Human Skin: Clinical and Molecular Evidence," https://www.ncbi.nlm.nih.gov, https://www.ncbi. nlm.nih.gov/pubmed/26492562, (2019 September 17)

173 LTD, Versus Arthritis Trading, "Types of complementary treatments; Pine Bark Extracts," https://www.versusarthritis.org, https://www. versusarthritis.org/about-arthritis/complementary-and-alternative-treatments/types-of-complementary-treatments/pine-bark-extracts/, (2019 July 17)

174 Fine AM, "Oligomeric proanthocyanidin complexes: history, structure, and phytopharmaceutical applications," https://www.ncbi.nlm.nih.gov. https://www.ncbi.nlm.nih.gov/pubmed/10767669, (2019 April 11)

175 Elsas SM, Rossi DJ, Raber J, White G, Seeley CA, Gregory WL, Mohr C, Pfankuch T, Soumyanath A., "Passiflora incarnata L. (Passionflower) extracts elicit GABA currents in hippocampal neurons in vitro, and show

anxiogenic and anticonvulsant effects in vivo, varying with extraction method," https://www.ncbi.nlm.nih.gov, https://www.ncbi.nlm.nih.gov/pmc/articles/PMC2941540/, (2019 September 17)

176 Hur MH, Yang YS, Lee MS, "Aromatherapy massage affects menopausal symptoms in Korean climacteric women: a pilot-controlled clinical trial," https://www.ncbi.nlm.nih.gov, https://www.ncbi.nlm.nih.gov/pmc/articles/PMC2529395/, (2018 November 18)

177 Limited, IndiaMART, "Parsley Essential Oils," https://www.indiaessentialoils.com, https://www.indiaessentialoils.com/parsley-seed-oil.html, (2019 September 14)

178 Benford Mafuvadze, Indira Benakanakere, Franklin R. López Pérez, Cynthia Besch-Williford, Mark R. Ellersieck, and Salman M. Hyder, "Apigenin Prevents Development of Medroxyprogesterone Acetate-Accelerated 7,12-Dimethylbenz(a)anthracene-Induced Mammary Tumors in Sprague–Dawley Rats," https://www.bibletecapleyades.net, https://www.bibliotecapleyades.net/archivos_pdf/apigenin-prevents-cancer-parsley.pdf, (2019 August 10)

179 Wiki, Cluefinders, "Tannin," https://cluefinders.fandom.com, https://cluefinders.fandom.com/wiki/Tannin, (2019 August 19)

180 LLC, Webmd, "Quercetin," https://www.webmd.com, https://www.webmd.com/vitamins/ai/ingredientmono-294/quercetin, (2019 May 14)

181 LLC, Paleo Leap, "The Health Benefits of Butyrate: Meet The Anti-Inflammatory Fat," https://paleoleap.com, https://paleoleap.com/butyrate-anti-inflammatory-fat/, (2018 March 15)

182 The George Mateljan Foundation, "What's New and Beneficial about Raspberries," http://www.whfoods.com/index.php http://www.whfoods.com/genpage.php?tname=foodspice&dbid=39, (2019 February 18)

183 Patel, Kamal, "Rose Hips," https://examine.com.https://examine.com/supplements/rose-hip/, (2019 July 7)

184 India Today, "Mooli for winters: 5 health benefits of radishes you shouldn't be deprived of," https://www.indiatoday.in, https://www.indiatoday.in/lifestyle/health/story/mooli-radish-health-benefits-winter-veggie-india-digestion-blood-pressure-lifest-1117051-2017-12-27, (2019 May 11)

[185] Med-Health, "Health benefit of Radishes," http://www.med-health.net. http://www.med-health.net/Health-Benefits-Of-Radishes.html, (2019 May 11)

[186] Panahi Y., Taghizadeh M, Marzony ET, Sahebkar A., "Rosemary oil vs minoxidil 2% for the treatment of androgenetic alopecia: a randomized comparative trial," http://europepmc.org, http://europepmc.org/abstract/med/25842469, (2019 January 11)

[187] SimonaBirtiÄ‡, PierreDussort, FranÃ§ois-XavierPierre, Antoine C.Bily, MarcRoller, "Applications of Carnosic Acid," https://agscientific.com https://agscientific.com/blog/2017/08/applications-of-carnosic-acid/, (2018 November 7)

[188] Margot Loussouarn, Anja Krieger-Liszkay,Ljubica Svilar, Antoine Bily, Simona Birtić, and Michel Havaux, "Carnosic Acid and Carnosol, Two Major Antioxidants of Rosemary, Act through Different Mechanisms," https://www.ncbi.nlm.nih.gov/, https://www.ncbi.nlm.nih.gov/pmc/articles/PMC5664485/, (2019 January 12).

[189] Elsevier B.V, "Cholorectic" https://www.sciencedirect.com, https://www.sciencedirect.com/topics/medicine-and-dentistry/choleretic, (2019 March 3)

[190] Moss M, Cook J, Wesnes K, Duckett P, "Aromas of rosemary and lavender essential oils differentially affect cognition and mood in healthy adults," https://www.ncbi.nlm.nih.gov, https://www.ncbi.nlm.nih.gov/pubmed/12690999, (2018 November 16)

[191] Raman, Ryan, "What is quercertin? Benefits, Foods, Dosage and Side effects," https://www.healthline.com, https://www.healthline.com/nutrition/quercetin#what-it-is, (2018, March 13)

[192] de la Lastra CA, Villegas I., "Resveratrol as an anti-inflammatory and anti-aging agent: mechanisms and clinical implications," https://www.ncbi.nlm.nih.gov/, https://www.ncbi.nlm.nih.gov/pubmed/15832402, (2019 July 10)

[193] Kwok Tung Lu, Robin Y. Y. Chiou, Li Ging Chen, Ming Hsiang Chen, Wan Ting Tseng, Hsiang Tsang Hsieh, Yi Ling Yang, "Neuroprotective Effects of Resveratrol on Cerebral Ischemia-Induced Neuron Loss Mediated by Free Radical Scavenging and Cerebral Blood Flow

Elevation," https://pubs.acs.org/, https://pubs.acs.org/doi/abs/10.1021/jf053011q, (2019 June 17)

[194] Burgess, Lana, "What are phytoestrogens? Benefits and foods," www.medicalnewstoday.com, https://www.medicalnewstoday.com/articles/320630.php, (2019 July 12)

[195] Soltani M, Khosravi AR, Asadi F, Shokri H., "Evaluation of protective efficacy of Spirulina platensis in Balb/C mice with candidiasis," https://www.ncbi.nlm.nih.gov,____https://www.ncbi.nlm.nih.gov/pubmed/23518167, (2019 March 3)

[196] Karkos PD, Leong SC, Karkos CD, Sivaji N, Assimakopoulos DA, "Spirulina in clinical practice: evidence-based human applications," https://www.ncbi.nlm.nih.gov,__https://www.ncbi.nlm.nih.gov/pmc/articles/PMC3136577/, (2019 March 6)

[197] Cheong SH, Kim MY, Sok DE, Hwang SY, Kim JH, Kim HR, Lee JH, Kim YB, Kim MR, "Spirulina prevents atherosclerosis by reducing hypercholesterolemia in rabbits fed a high-cholesterol diet," https://www.ncbi.nlm.nih.gov, https://www.ncbi.nlm.nih.gov/pubmed/20354344, (2019 March 6).

[198] Misbahuddin M, Islam AZ, Khandker S, Ifthaker-Al-Mahmud, Islam N, Anjumanara, "Efficacy of spirulina extract plus zinc in patients of chronic arsenic poisoning: a randomized placebo-controlled study," https://www.ncbi.nlm.nih.gov, https://www.ncbi.nlm.nih.gov/pubmed/16615668, (2019 March 5)

[199] Koníčková R, Vaňková K, Vaníková J, Váňová K, Muchová L, Subhanová I, Zadinová M, Zelenka J, Dvořák A, Kolář M, Strnad H, Rimpelová S, Ruml T, J Wong R, Vítek L., "Anti-cancer effects of blue-green alga Spirulina platensis, a natural source of bilirubin-like tetrapyrrolic compounds," https://www.ncbi.nlm.nih.gov, https://www.ncbi.nlm.nih.gov/pubmed/24552870, (2019 March 2)

[200] Healthline Media, "7 Surprising health benefits of eating seaweed," https://www.healthline.com, https://www.healthline.com/nutrition/benefits-of-seaweed#section4, (2019 March 18)

[201] Mourouzis I, Politi E, Pantos C., "Thyroid hormone and tissue repair: new tricks for an old hormone?" https://www.ncbi.nlm.nih.gov, https://www.ncbi.nlm.nih.gov/pmc/articles/PMC3596953/, (2019 March 13)

202 Maeda H, Hosokawa M, Sashima T, Murakami-Funayama K, Miyashita K., "Anti-obesity and anti-diabetic effects of fucoxanthin on diet-induced obesity conditions in a murine model," https://www.ncbi.nlm.nih.gov, https://www.ncbi.nlm.nih.gov/pubmed/21475918, (2019 March 11)

203 Masakazu Murata, Oxford AcademicGoogle ScholarKenji Ishihara, Oxford AcademicGoogle ScholarHiroaki Saito, "Hepatic Fatty Acid Oxidation Enzyme Activities are Stimulated in Rats Fed the Brown Seaweed," https://academic.oup.com, https://academic.oup.com/jn/article/129/1/146/4723215, (2019 March 17)

204 Jahnen-Dechent W, Ketteler M., "Magnesium basics," https://www.ncbi.nlm.nih.gov, https://www.ncbi.nlm.nih.gov/pmc/articles/PMC4455825/, (2019 March 29)

205 Dinan L., "The Karlson Lecture. Phytoecdysteroids: what use are they?" https://www.ncbi.nlm.nih.gov, https://www.ncbi.nlm.nih.gov/pubmed/19771554, (2019 March 25)

206 Wang Y, Chang CF, Chou J, Chen HL, Deng X, Harvey BK, Cadet JL, Bickford PC, "Dietary supplementation with blueberries, spinach, or spirulina reduces ischemic brain damage," https://www.ncbi.nlm.nih.gov, https://www.ncbi.nlm.nih.gov/pubmed/15817266, (2019 March 29)

207 Post RE, Mainous AG 3rd, King DE, Simpson KN. "Dietary fiber for the treatment of type 2 diabetes mellitus: a meta-analysis," https://www.ncbi.nlm.nih.gov, https://www.ncbi.nlm.nih.gov/pubmed/22218620, (2019 March 25)

208 Erlinger TP, Guallar E, Miller ER 3rd, Stolzenberg-Solomon R, Appel LJ, "Relationship between systemic markers of inflammation and serum beta-carotene levels," https://www.ncbi.nlm.nih.gov, https://www.ncbi.nlm.nih.gov/pubmed/11493133, (2019 March 24)

209 Stephensen CB, "Vitamin A, infection and immune function," https://www.ncbi.nlm.nih.gov, https://www.ncbi.nlm.nih.gov/pubmed/11375434, (2019 March 28)

210 Roberts RL, Green J, Lewis B., "Lutein and zeaxanthin in eye and skin health," https://www.ncbi.nlm.nih.gov, https://www.ncbi.nlm.nih.gov/pubmed/19168000, (2019 March 24)

211 Porrini M, Riso P, Oriani G. "Spinach and tomato consumption increases lymphocyte DNA resistance to oxidative stress but this is not

related to cell carotenoid concentrations," https://www.ncbi.nlm.nih.gov, https://www.ncbi.nlm.nih.gov/pubmed/12111045, (2019 March 26).

[212] Carr AC, Maggini S., "Vitamin C and Immune Function," https://www. ncbi.nlm.nih.gov,_https://www.ncbi.nlm.nih.gov/pubmed/29099763, (2019 March 28)

[213] Sankar D, Rao MR, Sambandam G, Pugalendi KV, "Effect of sesame oil on diuretics or Beta-blockers in the modulation of blood pressure, anthropometry, lipid profile, and redox status," https://www.ncbi.nlm. nih.gov, https://www.ncbi.nlm.nih.gov/pmc/articles/PMC1942178/, (2019 April 3)

[214] Wu WH, Kang YP, Wang NH, Jou HJ, Wang TA, "Sesame ingestion affects sex hormones, antioxidant status, and blood lipids in postmenopausal women," https://www.ncbi.nlm.nih.gov, https://www. ncbi.nlm.nih.gov/pubmed/16614415, (2019 April 3)

[215] McCann SE, Hootman KC, Weaver AM, Thompson LU, Morrison C, Hwang H, Edge SB, Ambrosone CB, Horvath PJ, Kulkarni SA, "Dietary intakes of total and specific lignans are associated with clinical breast tumor characteristics," https://www.ncbi.nlm.nih.gov, https://www.ncbi. nlm.nih.gov/pubmed/22113872, (2019 April 3)

[216] Fukumitsu S, Aida K, Shimizu H, Toyoda K., "Flaxseed lignan lowers blood cholesterol and decreases liver disease risk factors in moderately hypercholesterolemic men," https://www.ncbi.nlm.nih.gov, https://www. ncbi.nlm.nih.gov/pubmed/20797475, (2019 April 3)

[217] Pfeuffer M, Fielitz K, Laue C, Winkler P, Rubin D, Helwig U, Giller K, Kammann J, Schwedhelm E, Böger RH, Bub A, Bell D, Schrezenmeir J," CLA does not impair endothelial function and decreases body weight as compared with safflower oil in overweight and obese male subjects," https://www.ncbi.nlm.nih.gov, https://www.ncbi.nlm.nih.gov/ pubmed/21697535, (2019 April 4)

[218] Keen MA, Hassan I., "Vitamin E in dermatology," https://www.ncbi.nlm. nih.gov,_https://www.ncbi.nlm.nih.gov/pmc/articles/PMC4976416/, (2019 April 4)

[219] ScienceDirect, "Crocin," https://www.sciencedirect.com, https://www. sciencedirect.com/topics/neuroscience/crocin, (2019 March 15)

[220] Modabbernia A, Sohrabi H, Nasehi AA, Raisi F, Saroukhani S, Jamshidi A, Tabrizi M, Ashrafi M, Akhondzadeh S., "Effect of saffron on fluoxetine-induced sexual impairment in men: randomized double-blind placebo-controlled trial," https://www.ncbi.nlm.nih.gov, https://www.ncbi.nlm.nih.gov/pubmed/22552758, (2019 March 15)

[221] Hausenblas HA, Saha D, Dubyak PJ, Anton SD, "Saffron (Crocus sativus L.) and major depressive disorder: a meta-analysis of randomized clinical trials," https://www.ncbi.nlm.nih.gov, https://www.ncbi.nlm.nih.gov/pubmed/24299602, (2019 March 15)

[222] A DM, K S, A D, Sattar K., "Epidemiology of Premenstrual Syndrome (PMS)-A Systematic Review and Meta-Analysis Study," https://www.ncbi.nlm.nih.gov, https://www.ncbi.nlm.nih.gov/pubmed/24701496, (2019 March 15),

[223] Sá CM, Ramos AA, Azevedo MF, Lima CF, Fernandes-Ferreira M, Pereira-Wilson C., "Sage tea drinking improves lipid profile and antioxidant defenses in humans," https://www.ncbi.nlm.nih.gov, https://www.ncbi.nlm.nih.gov/pubmed/19865527, (2019 March 29)

[224] Beheshti-Rouy M, Azarsina M, Rezaie-Soufi L, Alikhani MY, Roshanaie G, Komaki S., "The antibacterial effect of sage extract (Salvia officinalis) mouthwash against Streptococcus mutans in dental plaque: a randomized clinical trial," https://www.ncbi.nlm.nih.gov, https://www.ncbi.nlm.nih.gov/pubmed/26668706, (2019 March 29)

[225] Akhondzadeh S, Noroozian M, Mohammadi M, Ohadinia S, Jamshidi AH, Khani M., "Salvia officinalis extract in the treatment of patients with mild to moderate Alzheimer's disease: a double blind, randomized and placebo-controlled trial," https://www.ncbi.nlm.nih.gov, https://www.ncbi.nlm.nih.gov/pubmed/12605619, (2019 March 29)

[226] Stremmel W, Gauss A., "Lecithin as a therapeutic agent in ulcerative colitis," https://www.ncbi.nlm.nih.gov, https://www.ncbi.nlm.nih.gov/pubmed/24246994, (2019 April 11)

[227] Lavigne V, Gleberzon BJ, "Ultrasound as a treatment of mammary blocked duct among 25 postpartum lactating women: a retrospective case series," https://www.ncbi.nlm.nih.gov, https://www.ncbi.nlm.nih.gov/pmc/articles/PMC3437340/, (2019 April 10)

228 Cox, Lauren, "What is Stevia?" https://www.livescience.com, https://www.livescience.com/39601-stevia-facts-safety.html, (2019 April 11)

229 Paul S, Sengupta S, Bandyopadhyay TK, Bhattacharyya A., "Stevioside induced ROS-mediated apoptosis through mitochondrial pathway in human breast cancer cell line MCF-7," https://www.ncbi.nlm.nih.gov, https://www.ncbi.nlm.nih.gov/pubmed/23061910, (2019 April 11)

230 Chatsudthipong V, Muanprasat C., "Stevioside and related compounds: therapeutic benefits beyond sweetness," https://www.ncbi.nlm.nih.gov, https://www.ncbi.nlm.nih.gov/pubmed/19000919, (2019 April 11)

231 LLC, Webmd, "Stoneroot," https://www.webmd.com, https://www.webmd.com/vitamins/ai/ingredientmono-89/stone-root, (2019 April 19)

232 Wholistic Matters, "Collinsonia Root: A Remedy Rooted in American History," https://wholisticmatters.com, https://wholisticmatters.com/collinsonia-root-a-remedy-rooted-in-american-history/, (2019 April 11)

233 Renner B, Ahne G, Grosan E, Kettenmann B, Kobal G, Shephard A., "Tonic stimulation of the pharyngeal mucosa causes pain and a reversible increase of inflammatory mediators," https://www.ncbi.nlm.nih.gov, https://www.ncbi.nlm.nih.gov/pubmed/24037371, (2019 April 11)

234 Pöldinger W., "History of St. John's wort," https://www.ncbi.nlm.nih.gov, https://www.ncbi.nlm.nih.gov/pubmed/11155493, (2019 May 14)

235 Ng QX, Venkatanarayanan N, Ho CY, "Clinical use of Hypericum perforatum (St John's wort) in depression: A meta-analysis," https://www.ncbi.nlm.nih.gov, https://www.ncbi.nlm.nih.gov/pubmed/28064110, (2019 May 14)

236 Grube B, Walper A, Wheatley D., "St. John's Wort extract: efficacy for menopausal symptoms of psychological origin," https://www.ncbi.nlm.nih.gov, https://www.ncbi.nlm.nih.gov/pubmed/10623319, (2019 May 17)

237 Martínez-Poveda B, Quesada AR, Medina MA, "Hyperforin, a bio-active compound of St. John's wort, is a new inhibitor of angiogenesis targeting several key steps of the process," https://www.ncbi.nlm.nih.gov, https://www.ncbi.nlm.nih.gov/pubmed/15981212, (2019 May 14)

238 Schempp CM, Windeck T, Hezel S, Simon JC, "Topical treatment of atopic dermatitis with St. John's wort cream—a randomized, placebo controlled, double blind half-side comparison," https://www.ncbi.nlm.

nih.gov, https://www.ncbi.nlm.nih.gov/pubmed/12807340, (2019 May 17)

239   Wilt Timothy; Ishani Areef, Gerold Stark, "Saw Palmetto Extracts for Treatment of Benign Prostatic Hyperplasia," https://jamanetwork.com, https://jamanetwork.com/journals/jama/article-abstract/188142?resultClick=1, (2019 May 18)

240   Prager N, Bickett K, French N, Marcovici G., "A randomized, double-blind, placebo-controlled trial to determine the effectiveness of botanically derived inhibitors of 5-alpha-reductase in the treatment of androgenetic alopecia," https://www.ncbi.nlm.nih.gov, https://www.ncbi.nlm.nih.gov/pubmed/12006122, (2019 May 18)

241   Darrow, J; Cranwell, W. "Everything you need to know about DHT," https://www.medicalnewstoday.com, https://www.medicalnewstoday.com/articles/68082.php, (2019 May 16)

242   Suter A, Saller R, Riedi E, Heinrich M., "Improving BPH symptoms and sexual dysfunctions with a saw palmetto preparation? Results from a pilot trial," https://www.ncbi.nlm.nih.gov, https://www.ncbi.nlm.nih.gov/pubmed/22522969, (2019 May 19)

243   Padayatty SJ, Katz A, Wang Y, Eck P, Kwon O, Lee JH, Chen S, Corpe C, Dutta A, Dutta SK, Levine M., "Vitamin C as an antioxidant: evaluation of its role in disease prevention," https://www.ncbi.nlm.nih.gov, https://www.ncbi.nlm.nih.gov/pubmed/12569111, (2019 May 23)

244   Anderson JW, Baird P, Davis RH Jr, Ferreri S, Knudtson M, Koraym A, Waters V, Williams CL, "Health benefits of dietary fiber," https://www.ncbi.nlm.nih.gov, https://www.ncbi.nlm.nih.gov/pubmed/19335713, (2019 May 23)

245   LLC, Webmd, "Quercetin," https://www.webmd.com. https://www.webmd.com/vitamins-and-supplements/quercetin-uses-and-risks#1, (2019 May 23)

246   Anderson JW, Baird P, Davis RH Jr, Ferreri S, Knudtson M, Koraym A, Waters V, Williams CL, "Health benefits of dietary fiber," https://www.ncbi.nlm.nih.gov, https://www.ncbi.nlm.nih.gov/pubmed/19335713, (2019 May 23)

247   Wintergerst ES, Maggini S, Hornig DH, "Immune-enhancing role of vitamin C and zinc and effect on clinical conditions," https://www.ncbi.

nlm.nih.gov, https://www.ncbi.nlm.nih.gov/pubmed/16373990, (2019 May 23)

248 LLC, Webmd, "Lycopene," https://webmd.com, https://www.webmd.com/vitamins/ai/ingredientmono-554/lycopene, (2019 March 6)

249 Giovannucci E., "A review of epidemiologic studies of tomatoes, lycopene, and prostate cancer," https://www.ncbi.nlm.nih.gov, https://www.ncbi.nlm.nih.gov/pubmed/12424325, (2019 September 6)

250 LLC, Webmd, "Lutein," https://www.webmd.com, https://www.webmd.com/vitamins/ai/ingredientmono-754/lutein, (2019 September 5)

251 Chambial S, Dwivedi S, Shukla KK, John PJ, Sharma P., "Vitamin C in disease prevention and cure: an overview," https://www.ncbi.nlm.nih.gov, https://www.ncbi.nlm.nih.gov/pmc/articles/PMC3783921/, (2019 September 5)

252 Berkheiser, Kaitlyn, "Tangerines vs. Oranges: How Are They Different?"

253 https://www.healthline.com, https://www.healthline.com/nutrition/tangerine-vs-orange#bottom-line, (2019 September 6)

254 Kuru, Pinar, "Tamarindus indica and its health-related effects," https://www.sciencedirect.com, https://www.sciencedirect.com/science/article/pii/S2221169115300885#bib12, (2019 September 6)

255 Sundaram MS, Hemshekhar M, Santhosh MS, Paul M, Sunitha K, Thushara RM, NaveenKumar SK, Naveen S, Devaraja S, Rangappa KS, Kemparaju K, Girish KS, "Tamarind Seed (Tamarindus indica) Extract Ameliorates Adjuvant-Induced Arthritis via Regulating the Mediators of Cartilage/Bone Degeneration, Inflammation and Oxidative Stress," https://www.ncbi.nlm.nih.gov, https://www.ncbi.nlm.nih.gov/pmc/articles/PMC4461917/, (2019 September 6)

256 Jahnen-Dechent W, Ketteler M., "Magnesium basics," https://www.ncbi.nlm.nih.gov, https://www.ncbi.nlm.nih.gov/pmc/articles/PMC4455825/, (2019 September 6)

257 Raeisi M., Tajik H., Razavi RS, Maham M., Moradi M., Hajimohammadi B., Naghili H., Hashemi M., Mehdizadeh T., "Essential oil of tarragon (Artemisia dracunculus) antibacterial activity on Staphylococcus aureus and Escherichia coli in culture media and Iranian white cheese," https://www.ncbi.nlm.nih.gov, https://www.ncbi.nlm.nih.gov/pmc/articles/PMC3391558/, (2019 September 6)

258 Xu JS, Li Y, Cao X, Cui Y., "The effect of eugenol on the cariogenic properties of Streptococcus mutans and dental caries development in rats," https://www.ncbi.nlm.nih.gov, https://www.ncbi.nlm.nih.gov/pmc/articles/PMC3702691/, (2019 September 6)

259 Schnitzler P, Schön K, Reichling J., "Antiviral activity of Australian tea tree oil and eucalyptus oil against herpes simplex virus in cell culture," https://www.ncbi.nlm.nih.gov, https://www.ncbi.nlm.nih.gov/pubmed/11338678, (2019 September 6)

260 Carson CF, Hammer KA, Riley TV, "Melaleuca alternifolia (Tea Tree) oil: a review of antimicrobial and other medicinal properties," https://www.ncbi.nlm.nih.gov, https://www.ncbi.nlm.nih.gov/pmc/articles/PMC1360273/, (2019 September 6)

261 Foundation Matelijan George The, "Thyme," http://www.whfoods.com, http://www.whfoods.com/genpage.php?tname=foodspice&dbid=77#healthbenefits, (2019 September 8)

262 Sienkiewicz M., Łysakowska M., Ciećwierz J., Denys P., Kowalczyk E., "Antibacterial activity of thyme and lavender essential oils," https://www.ncbi.nlm.nih.gov, https://www.ncbi.nlm.nih.gov/pubmed/22313307, (2019 September 8)

263 Nostro A, Papalia T., "Antimicrobial activity of carvacrol: current progress and future prospectives," https://www.ncbi.nlm.nih.gov, https://www.ncbi.nlm.nih.gov/pubmed/22044355, (2018 April 11)

264 Group, Dr. Edward, "What Is Carvacrol? 8 Facts to Know," https://www.globalhealingcenter.com, https://www.globalhealingcenter.com/natural-health/what-is-carvacrol-8-facts-to-know/, (2019 September 8)

265 Fan K, Li X, Cao Y, Qi H, Li L, Zhang Q, Sun H., "Carvacrol inhibits proliferation and induces apoptosis in human colon cancer cells," https://www.ncbi.nlm.nih.gov, https://www.ncbi.nlm.nih.gov/pubmed/26214321, (2019 September 8)

266 Margherita Zotti, Marilena Colaianna, Maria Grazia Morgese, Paolo Tucci, Stefania Schiavone, Pinarosa Avato Luigia Trabace,, "Carvacrol: From Ancient Flavoring to Neuromodulatory Agent," https://www.mdpi.com, https://www.mdpi.com/1420-3049/18/6/6161, (2019 September 8)

267 Shoba G., Joy D., Joseph T., Majeed M., Rajendran R., Srinivas PS, "Influence of piperine on the pharmacokinetics of curcumin in animals

and human volunteers," https://www.ncbi.nlm.nih.gov, https://www.ncbi.nlm.nih.gov/pubmed/9619120, (2019 September 16)

[268] Kim T, Davis J, Zhang AJ, He X, Mathews ST, "Curcumin activates AMPK and suppresses gluconeogenic gene expression in hepatoma cells," https://www.ncbi.nlm.nih.gov, https://www.ncbi.nlm.nih.gov/pubmed/19665995, (2019 September 16)

[269] Marín YE, Wall BA, Wang S, Namkoong J, Martino JJ, Suh J, Lee HJ, Rabson AB, Yang CS, Chen S, Ryu JH, "Curcumin downregulates the constitutive activity of NF-kappaB and induces apoptosis in novel mouse melanoma cells," https://www.ncbi.nlm.nih.gov, https://www.ncbi.nlm.nih.gov/pubmed/17885582, (2019 September 16)

[270] Singh S, Aggarwal Bharat, "Activation of Transcription Factor NF-κB Is Suppressed by Curcumin (Diferuloylmethane)," http://www.jbc.org. http://www.jbc.org/content/270/42/24995.full, (2019 September 16)

[271] Di Pierro F, Bressan A, Ranaldi D, Rapacioli G, Giacomelli L, Bertuccioli A., "Potential role of bioavailable curcumin in weight loss and omental adipose tissue decrease: preliminary data of a randomized, controlled trial in overweight people with metabolic syndrome. Preliminary study," https://www.ncbi.nlm.nih.gov, https://www.ncbi.nlm.nih.gov/pubmed/26592847, (2019 September 16)

[272] Ramírez-Tortosa MC, Mesa MD, Aguilera MC, Quiles JL, Baró L, Ramirez-Tortosa CL, Martinez-Victoria E, Gil A., "Oral administration of a turmeric extract inhibits LDL oxidation and has hypocholesterolemic effects in rabbits with experimental atherosclerosis," https://www.ncbi.nlm.nih.gov, https://www.ncbi.nlm.nih.gov/pubmed/10559523, (2019 September 16)

[273] Kulkarni S.K., Dhir Ashish, Akula Kiran, "Potentials of Curcumin as an Antidepressant," https://www.hindawi.com, https://www.hindawi.com/journals/tswj/2009/624894/abs/, (2019 September 16)

[274] Sanmukhani J, Satodia V, Trivedi J, Patel T, Tiwari D, Panchal B, Goel A, Tripathi CB, "Efficacy and safety of curcumin in major depressive disorder: a randomized controlled trial," https://www.ncbi.nlm.nih.gov, https://www.ncbi.nlm.nih.gov/pubmed/23832433, (2019 September 16)

275 Brazier, Yvette, "What is thiamine, or vitamin B1?" https://www.medicalnewstoday.com, https://www.medicalnewstoday.com/articles/219545.php, (2019 September 18)

276 Wilson Sue, Gardiner, Anne, "Pectin and Partners for Perfect Preserves," https://www.exploratorium.edu, https://www.exploratorium.edu/cooking/icooks/article_6-03.html, (2019 June 22)

277 Shyamala BN, Naidu MM, Sulochanamma G, Srinivas P., "Studies on the antioxidant activities of natural vanilla extract and its constituent compounds through in vitro models," https://www.ncbi.nlm.nih.gov, https://www.ncbi.nlm.nih.gov/pubmed/17715988, (2019 September 19)

278 Ghaemi EO, Khorshidi D, Moradi A, Seifi A, Mazendrani M, Bazouri M, Mansourian AR, "The efficacy of ethanolic extract of Lemon verbena on the skin infection due to Staphylococcus aureus in an animal model," https://www.ncbi.nlm.nih.gov, https://www.ncbi.nlm.nih.gov/pubmed/19090293, (2019 March 11)

279 Hasler G, van der Veen JW, Grillon C, Drevets WC, Shen J., "Effect of acute psychological stress on prefrontal GABA concentration determined by proton magnetic resonance spectroscopy," https://www.ncbi.nlm.nih.gov, https://www.ncbi.nlm.nih.gov/pubmed/20634372, (2019 March 9)

280 Collins JK, Wu G, Perkins-Veazie P, Spears K, Claypool PL, Baker RA, Clevidence BA, "Watermelon consumption increases plasma arginine concentrations in adults," https://www.ncbi.nlm.nih.gov, https://www.ncbi.nlm.nih.gov/pubmed/17352962, (2019 October 19)

281 Goldman, Rena, Watson, Kathryn, "Willow Bark: Nature's Aspirin?" https://www.healthline.com, https://www.healthline.com/health/willow-bark-natures-aspirin, (2019 September 13)

282 Sethi J, Yadav M, Dahiya K, Sood S, Singh V, Bhattacharya SB, "Antioxidant effect of Triticum aestivium (wheat grass) in high-fat diet-induced oxidative stress in rabbits," https://www.ncbi.nlm.nih.gov, https://www.ncbi.nlm.nih.gov/pubmed/20508870, (2019 October 24)

283 Allen Suzanne, PhD Boskey Elizabeth, Cherney Kristeen, "Acidosis," https://www.healthline.com, https://www.healthline.com/health/acidosis, (2018 May 3)

284   RD Link, Rachael, "10 Proven Probiotic Yogurt Benefits & Nutrition Facts," www.draxe.com, https://draxe.com/nutrition/probiotic-yogurt/, (2019 November 1)

285   Cerhan JR, Saag KG, Merlino LA, Mikuls TR, Criswell LA, "Antioxidant micronutrients and risk of rheumatoid arthritis in a cohort of older women," https://www.ncbi.nlm.nih.gov, https://www.ncbi.nlm.nih.gov/pubmed/12578805, (2019 January 17)

286   Dawid-Pać R., "Medicinal plants used in treatment of inflammatory skin diseases," https://www.ncbi.nlm.nih.gov, https://www.ncbi.nlm.nih.gov/pmc/articles/PMC3834722/, (2019 March 12)

287   AskMayoExpert, "Mastitis," https://www.mayoclinic.org, https://www.mayoclinic.org/diseases-conditions/mastitis/symptoms-causes/syc-20374829, (2019 July 16)

288   Miller FM, Chow LM, "Yarrow: The Healing Herb of Achilles," https://sites.evergreen.edu, https://sites.evergreen.edu/plantchemeco/yarrow-the-healing-herb-of-achilles/, (2019 October 29)

289   González-Verdejo CI, Obrero Á, Román B, Gómez P.," Expression Profile of Carotenoid Cleavage Dioxygenase Genes in Summer Squash (Cucurbita pepo L.)," https://www.ncbi.nlm.nih.gov, https://www.ncbi.nlm.nih.gov/pubmed/25861766, (2019 October 21)

290   Piche T., "Tight junctions and IBS—the link between epithelial permeability, low-grade inflammation, and symptom generation?" https://www.ncbi.nlm.nih.gov, https://www.ncbi.nlm.nih.gov/pubmed/24548256, (2019 October 21)

291   Brouns F., Theuwissen E., Adam A., Bell M., Berger A., Mensink RP, "Cholesterol-lowering properties of different pectin types in mildly hyper-cholesterolemic men and women," https://www.ncbi.nlm.nih.gov, https://www.ncbi.nlm.nih.gov/pubmed/22190137, (2019 October 21)

292   American Pregnancy Association, "Roles of Vitamin B in pregnancy," https://americanpregnancy.org, https://americanpregnancy.org/pregnancy-health/vitamin-b-pregnancy/, (2019 October 21)

293   Mares, Julie, "Lutein and Zeaxanthin Isomers in Eye Health and Disease," https://www.ncbi.nlm.nih.gov/pmc/articles/PMC5611842/, https://www.ncbi.nlm.nih.gov, https://www.ncbi.nlm.nih.gov/pmc/articles/PMC5611842/, (2019 October 21)

INDEX

A

Acetylcholine, 215, 217
acid reflux, 9, 13, 78, 251, 266
acne, 10, 13, 39, 54, 61, 86,
    96, 111–112, 132, 157,
    229, 233
acute dermatitis (eczema),
    5–6, 13–14, 75–76,
    102–103, 116–117,
    152–153, 176–177,
    213–214, 262–263
ADHD, 57
adipokine secretion, 29
adsorption, 46
alkaline food, 49
Alzheimer, 12, 36, 44–45,
    133, 215
amino acid L-tryptophan, 167
anti-aging treatment, 156
antifungal properties, 13, 26,
    79, 112, 233–234
anxiety, 25, 41, 72, 75,
    110–111, 129, 132, 134,
    144, 181, 220, 237, 244,
    246
Arsenic poisoning, 202–203
asthma, 5, 26, 30–31, 94, 136,
145, 182, 247
atherosclerosis, 3, 6, 29, 32,
    47, 81, 100, 130, 189, 199,
    202, 209, 224, 236–237
autoimmune diseases, 22
Azadirachtin, 148

B

bacillus subtilis, 234
bacterial infections, 32, 50, 96
bad acne, 39, 86
bad breath, 182, 233
bad cholesterol, 205–206,
    234, 237
bad coughs, 94
benign prostate hypertrophy
    (BPH), 222
beta-carotene, 8, 40, 45, 48,
    168, 172–173, 175, 184
blood sugar levels, 9, 15, 18,
    33, 46, 56, 68, 90, 98, 124,
    140–141, 181, 192, 224,
    240
bone pain, 53
brain's GABA (Gamma
    Amino- butyric acid), 246
breakdown of (ACH), 215
breast cancer, 16, 22, 46, 50,

53, 72, 87, 116, 178,
211–212, 218, 234
bronchitis, 80, 94, 136, 219,
231
bug bite, 10

C

Calcium channel blockers, 53
cancers, 2, 4, 20, 24, 31, 35,
46, 53, 58, 86–87, 120,
125, 161, 228, 236, 254
cardiovascular disease, 24, 40,
52, 202, 225
cardiovascular system, 5, 14,
35, 40, 87, 127
carotenoid crocin, 214
celiac disease, 81, 188
cell viability, 16
Charlie horse, 100, 252
chlorella, 59, 202
Cholesterol, 2, 4–5, 15–16,
23–27, 64–67, 151–152,
178, 205–206, 215, 228,
236–237, 264
chronic constipation, 209
chronic inflammation, 16, 23,
31–32, 38, 56, 121, 152,
163, 180, 194, 206,
213–215, 233, 245
circulation, 10, 50, 65, 70, 94,
127–128, 190, 199, 219,
250, 262
cirrhosis, 8, 19, 98, 142, 196

cold, 5, 13, 32–33, 35, 48, 60,
82, 86, 118–121, 155–156,
161, 176, 192, 209, 224,
258
cold sores, 35, 53, 129
congestive heart failure (CHF),
4
COPD, 94, 145
Crohn's disease, 53, 116, 189,
217

D

dark marks, 5–6, 132
dehydration, 54, 174, 250
Dementia, 12, 36, 44, 152,
155, 215
depression, 41, 57, 66, 71–72,
110, 134, 181, 214, 220,
237, 244
diabetes, 2, 4–5, 12, 23, 29,
46–48, 56–58, 87, 109,
150, 161, 185, 204,
224–226, 258
diarrhea, 15, 75, 99, 107, 109,
135, 178
digestion, 4, 13, 48, 56, 65,
78–79, 97, 111, 151, 168,
178, 192, 198, 205,
231–232, 258
dihydrotestosterone (DHT),
222
diverticulitis, 19, 35, 53, 190,
193, 198, 217, 225, 253

Diverticulosis, 19, 35, 65, 171, 209, 217, 225

dry skin, 110, 112, 195, 213

E

eczema, 26, 39, 72, 75, 80, 102, 110–112, 116, 137, 152, 160, 176, 181, 213, 220, 229, 233, 262

edema, 3, 30, 33, 131, 183, 244, 250

elderberries' anthocyanins, 33

epilepsy, 35, 66

Escherichia coli, 234

F

fat metabolism, 50

fatigue, 36, 72, 90, 155, 180, 220

fever, 10, 129, 132, 258, 261

flu, 5, 32, 75, 258

Folate, 3, 15, 19, 23, 37–39, 74, 101, 170, 182, 184, 193, 204, 228, 253, 264

frostbite, 13

fungi, 10, 50, 66, 163, 202, 234, 260

G

GABA levels, 181

gallbladder disease, 142

gamma linoleic acid (GLA), 102

gastroesophageal reflux disease (GERD), 9, 13, 55, 72, 78, 92, 96, 224, 251, 266

gastrointestinal diseases, 140

glucoraphanin, 30

glucosinolates, 22–23, 30, 121

glutathione levels, 12

gluten sensitive, 81

Gout, 37, 52

gut flora, 15, 24, 88, 117, 178, 202, 209

H

halitosis, 182, 233

hand eczema, 26

HDL, 9, 32, 67, 98, 103, 172, 202, 215, 234

headache, 75, 134, 225

heart disease, 4, 15–16, 20–25, 56–57, 65, 106, 130, 151–152, 175, 185, 213, 236, 250, 264

heartache, 134

herpes, 5, 13, 32, 53, 75, 129, 233, 241

high blood pressure (HBP), 4, 9, 15, 21, 26, 28, 51, 53, 89, 125, 135, 180–181, 211, 244, 264

high cholesterol, 4, 9, 16, 21, 26, 38, 41, 154, 158, 178, 185, 202, 206, 209, 228, 230, 236–237, 264 higher plasma HDL cholesterol, 215

human papilloma virus (HPV), 59, 241

hyperpigmentation, 86, 180, 182, 206, 229, 260

hypoglycemizing activity, 16

hypolipidemizing activity, 16

I

inflammation, 2, 5–6, 10, 22–23, 29–33, 47, 51–57, 72–73, 91–92, 136–137, 166–167, 208–209, 236, 254, 262, 266

influenza, 32

insomnia, 131, 181, 246

insulin sensitivity, 9, 23, 29, 90

iron deficient, 15, 18, 24, 126

irritable bowel syndrome (IBS), 2, 72, 94, 107, 116, 118, 120, 176, 189, 202, 217, 258, 264

irritation, 13, 33, 116, 120, 132, 219–220, 254

K

keratosis, 203

keto fans, 15

keto lifestyle, 226

kidney issues, 5

L

LDL levels, 98

leaky bowel syndrome, 53

leukemia, 53

lipid, 9, 29, 50–51, 66, 68, 74, 87, 131, 196, 211, 215, 254

liver cancer, 98

liver disease, 2, 98

liver failure, 98

low-carb dieters, 15

low-density lipoproteins (LDL), 9, 20, 67, 87, 103, 141, 154, 158, 161, 172, 202, 206, 215, 234, 236

lower blood pressure, 12, 19, 47, 53–54, 60, 67, 81, 98, 127, 154, 185, 189, 218

lower plasma LDL cholesterol, 215

lycopene, 59, 65, 86, 89, 228, 250

M

Macular degeneration, 7, 23, 40, 52, 73, 94, 150, 169, 175, 182, 184, 210, 228, 265

Manganese, 25, 35, 55, 70, 145, 158, 184, 188, 193, 206–207, 211, 253, 260

Mastitis, 262

melanosis, 203

metabolic syndrome, 87, 98, 107, 236

Metabolism, 29, 36, 39, 47, 50, 57, 71, 86, 93, 132, 170, 192, 198, 208, 264
minor inflammation, 13
mitochondria, 19, 29
MSRA, 27, 96
myrosinase, 30

N
Nasunin, 70
non-stop energy, 18

O
oily skin, 110, 112, 176
Osteopenia, 22, 57, 106, 116, 118, 158, 184, 193, 198, 208, 258
osteoporosis, 38, 57, 74, 106, 116, 118, 158, 162, 170, 184, 193, 204, 208, 258
oxidative stress, 6, 16, 22–23, 34–35, 47, 57, 90, 124, 132–133, 145, 208–210, 214–215, 254, 264

P
pancreatic beta cells, 5
Parkinson's disease, 2, 44
plant-based eater, 15
PMS'ing, 18
Polyacetylenes, 50
poor eyesight, 175
Postpartum depression, 134
prediabetic, 56, 74, 154

prostate cancer cells, 37
psoriasis, 72, 75, 102, 116, 213, 254

R
renal disease, 5
renin-angiotensin system, 211
rheumatoid arthritis, 22, 26, 260

S
Selenium, 39, 41, 253
severe cough, 131–132, 136
shigella sonnei, 234
sinus infection, 33, 37, 110, 176, 233
skin irritations, 116, 132, 254
sleep apnea, 96, 232
sleep deprivation, 111, 144
staphylococcus aureus, 27, 131, 234, 245
stomach ulcers, 13, 35, 137
stress, 2, 45, 47, 59–60, 79, 98, 109–111, 134, 137, 144, 154–156, 170, 231, 246
sulforaphane (SUL), 22, 30–31
swelling, 10, 33, 54, 72, 78, 109, 131, 167, 197, 214, 219, 233

T
tetrahydrocannabinol (THC), 102

treatment of alopecia, 196
tryptophan, 18, 167
type 2 diabetes, 4, 44, 46, 87,
191, 240, 258

U
ulcerative colitis, 80, 109, 131
ulcers, 13, 35, 50, 137, 178,
195, 206, 209, 224, 246
unnecessary toxins, 15, 27, 30,
106
unwanted blemishes, 110
unwanted weight gain, 27
upset stomach, 10, 15, 26, 55,
92, 106, 109, 131, 163,
178, 258
urinary tract infections (UTI),
3, 21, 50, 52, 55, 111, 155,
233, 241

V
varicose veins, 219
vegan, 6, 15, 41, 47, 74, 106,
124, 152, 158
vestibular nerve, 132
viral infections, 13, 53
vitamin B6, 3, 18, 37, 106,
140

W
weak immune system, 5, 27,
90, 241
wrinkles, 110, 125, 128, 140,
143, 169, 173, 190, 194,

206, 229, 251

Y
yeast infections, 75, 132, 202